The Vitality Diet: The Vegetarian/Vegan Anti-Inflammatory Diet & Recipe Book

The Vitality Diet: The Vegetarian/Vegan Anti-Inflammatory Diet & Recipe Book

THE SCIENCE-BASED WAY TO OVERCOME CHRONIC PAIN, DISEASE, AND WEIGHT GAIN, AND TO RESTORE YOUR BODY'S TOTAL HEALTH AND VITALITY

Sarah Grace Manski MS.

© 2017 Sarah Grace Manski MS. All rights reserved.

No part of this book may be reproduced in any written, electronic, recording, or photocopying without written permission of the publisher or author. The exception would be in the case of brief quotations embodied in the critical articles or reviews and pages where permission is specifically granted by the publisher or author.

Although every precaution has been taken to verify the accuracy of the information contained herein, the author and publisher assume no responsibility for any errors or omissions. No liability is assumed for damages that may result from the use of information contained within.

ISBN-13: 9781542531733
ISBN-10: 154253173X
Library of Congress Control Number: 2017900657
CreateSpace Independent Publishing Platform
North Charleston, South Carolina

Preface

Thank you for your interest in this book and in the anti-inflammatory diet. This book will introduce you to scientific research and health information that will help you improve your life. The anti-inflammatory diet is not a fad; it has been used by thousands of people for the last 30 years, helping them obtain their ideal bodies and increase their overall sense of well-being. More than just a diet, countering inflammation is also a lifestyle for vitality and happiness. The commitment it offers to healthy living and eating not only manages to establish a healthy weight, but also to fight or even avoid illness. This book contains recipes for breakfasts, lunches and dinners made with ingredients that are easily available. You will find these recipes quick and simple, with clear and concise cooking instructions. Enjoy life!

Vitality involves more than just eating right, so in this book I offer an overall approach to achieving vitality. Once you change your diet, you will immediately notice an increase in physical strength and mental vigor.

You probably know people who embody the concept of vitality. They're the people in your life with almost endless energy, the friends and family members that have passion and empathy. Being in their presence calms and energizes you—they just feel good to be around. Their enthusiasm for life rubs off on you. They just have something different, something special.

Where do these people get their vitality?

When we observe people who exude vitality, we see it in the way that they move and the way that they look. Their eyes glow, their skin radiates life, and they are always up for a challenge or an adventure. Because we see these very real physical characteristics, we often believe that they get their vitality from their health. While health is a part of vitality, it is by no means the only factor that contributes to this way of life. As you've probably observed, even those with ailments and illnesses can be incredibly vital.

Vitality is certainly enhanced by making the right choices and taking care of the body. Those who don't take care of their bodies are less likely to have this trait, but vitality may actually be the cause, and not the result, of better, healthier habits. Just getting healthy does not necessarily mean that you will gain vitality.

Are there habits that a person can practice to build their own vitality? Where does vitality originate, and if you lose it, where does it go? Are there habits that will make it more likely that your vitality will decrease?

To get to those questions, let's first ask another: What is vitality? Most cultures have some concept of vitality. We often think of it as a reservoir of energy and a resilience to stress and sadness. This same concept is embodied in the Eastern belief in "chi," or "prana." These words describe the life force that fuels both people and everything living in the world. It is both mental and physical.

Here in North America, we often think of vitality as something nice to have, but not a necessary part of life. In the East, vitality is an integral part of tradition and belief. It seeps into every aspect of life, from a person's environment, to their general attitude, to how honest they are, and how focused they are on a spiritual purpose.

When you visit a doctor in the West, they will evaluate you on your lack of illnesses. If your tests don't show that you have high blood pressure, heart disease, or other issues, they assume you are healthy. They are not concerned with whether or not your life has purpose, which is a major indicator of whether or not you also have vitality. You can be in perfect health and still not have vitality.

In Greek, there are two words that help us understand how health and vitality are connected. "Bios," which means life, and "zöe," which has to do with the "essence" of a person. Your bios is your health—your skin, organs, veins, cells, and natural processes. This is how we in the West usually determine health, by observing those processes, ignoring the "essence" altogether. In order to have vitality, we must care for the bios and the zöe. Without caring for the zöe, we are merely surviving. Tending to it brings us mental and physical satisfaction, which brings vitality.

In Okinawa, Japan, the average person lives seven years longer than the average person in the USA. In a relatively undeveloped portion of Sardinia, the rate of men reaching a hundred years old is ten times higher than in most developed countries. They also have lower rates of diabetes, cancers, and heart disease (the three most common serious maladies in the USA). Much of this difference can be attributed to the naturally anti-inflammatory diet that these people follow, but it is also important to acknowledge the lifestyle, not just the diet, in these regions of the world. In other cultures, finding purpose and living a balanced life, as well as having strong ties to the spiritual world and to your family and community are very important. They may be as important as diet to living a long life and developing and maintaining vitality.

Nonetheless, you may find it easier and quicker to alter your diet than to recreate your place in society. The good news is that an anti-inflammatory diet can take care of the health and wellness aspects of vitality. As your body heals and you lose weight, it will then be easier to find your life's purpose and to find satisfaction, and ultimately, vitality.

~ Sarah Grace Manski
Master of Science, Life Sciences Communication, UW Madison

p.s. - Obligatory legal disclaimer: This book is simply an introduction to the anti-inflammatory diet. This book is not intended to serve as a medical prescription or to replace the advice of your medical doctor. And please do speak with your primary care physician about what you read here!

Table of Contents

Preface · v

Foreword by Dr. Jill Stein, MD · xiii

Introduction · xix

Part 1: Understanding the Science · 1

Chapter 1   What is Inflammation? · 3

Chapter 2   What Inflammation Looks Like · 5

Chapter 3   Why Inflammation Makes You Fat · 6

Chapter 4   Why Inflammation Makes You Sick · 8

Chapter 5   Candida Yeast and Other Yeast Infections · · · · · · · · · · · · · · · · · · 14

Chapter 6   Before, We Had Little to Eat: An Evolutionary Explanation behind Our Cravings for Sugar and Fat · 16

Chapter 7   Gardening Your Gut: Clearing the Field and Planting What You Want · 20

Chapter 8	How to Listen to Your Body	22
Chapter 9	The Research Demonstrating the Benefits of an Anti-Inflammatory Vitality Diet	26

Part 2: Taking Action ... 37

Chapter 10	Foods that Heal, Foods that Hurt and Why	39
Chapter 11	Beginners Guide to the Anti-Inflammatory Diet: The Basics	44
Chapter 12	Great Salads are a Start	46
Chapter 13	Stay Hydrated and Restore Alkalinity to Your Body	49
Chapter 14	10 Easy Ways to Drink More Water for Weight Loss	51
Chapter 15	Detox Your Home and Throw The Poisons Out!	53
Chapter 16	Anti-Inflammatory Essentials: What You Should Always Have In Your Kitchen	58
Chapter 17	Pills and Supplements: What to Look For	60
Chapter 18	What Is The Difference Between Omega-3 And Omega-6?	62
Chapter 19	Research Shows You May Not Be Losing Weight Because You Need Vitamin D	64
Chapter 20	The Gym Isn't As Important As You Think It Is	66
Chapter 21	Stop Counting Calories! Why Calorie Counting Won't Help You Lose Weight	67

Part 3: The World and You		71
Chapter 22	If Slow is Good for Food, Why Not Medicine?	73
Chapter 23	Policies to Make the World a Healthful Planet	75
Chapter 24	Research Shows How Chiropractic Care Helps Weight Loss	76
Chapter 25	Inset by Eric F. Watts D.C.	78
Chapter 26	Maintaining a Positive Attitude	80
Chapter 27	10 Ways to Achieve Lasting Happiness	82
Chapter 28	Raising an Anti-Inflammatory Family in an "Inflammatory" World	84
Chapter 29	Animals and Inflammation: Why Anti-Inflammatory Should Also be Vegetarian or Vegan	87
Part 4: Anti-Inflammatory Meal Ideas		93
Chapter 1	Breakfast	95
Chapter 2	Snacks	138
Chapter 3	Lunch and Dinner	162
Chapter 4	Sweet Treats	261
Chapter 5	Whole Week Grocery Shopping	280

Foreword by Dr. Jill Stein, MD

As you're about to read, Sarah Manski's life changed when she started eating an anti-inflammatory diet of plant-based, fresh, unprocessed whole foods. Sarah effortlessly shed excess weight and experienced a dramatic increase in energy. Sarah's experience is not uncommon in the world of anti-inflammatory diets. Her Vitality Diet is a simple and alluring entry into the vibrant world of anti-inflammatory eating.

Anti-inflammatory diets are generally based on the widely accepted scientific principle that over-activity of the immune system is linked to a variety of modern diseases - from heart disease, obesity, diabetes, osteoporosis, rheumatoid arthritis and Alzheimer's to depression, insomnia and asthma. To various degrees, these diets reduce nutrients that ramp up the body's inflammatory response, and increase the nutrients that support an anti-inflammatory state of the immune system.

Diet, of course, is not the only driver of an overactive immune system. Exposure to air pollution and other environmentally introduced chemicals, a sedentary lifestyle, and psychosocial stress (induced by poverty, violence, homelessness, unemployment etc.) are all implicated. Among these factors, diet, in theory at least, is subject to individual control. Unfortunately, harmful government policies, bought through agribusiness campaign contributions and lobbyists, subsidize nutrient-poor industry food, and make healthy fresh fruits and vegetables less accessible and more expensive. So food is becoming less an individual choice, and more a matter of corrupt political forces. Knowing the health consequences of the food we eat allows us to optimize what choices we have, better protect our health, and fight more effectively for food justice and democracy.

Well Documented Health Benefits of the Best Known Anti-Inflammatory Diet

While there are many forms of the anti-inflammatory diet, the basic principles of these diets are similar to each other. The best known is perhaps the Mediterranean diet, which has been extensively researched and shown to have powerful health benefits across a broad spectrum of chronic disease. Like the Vitality Diet, the Mediterranean diet consists of fresh fruits and vegetables, legumes (such as lentils and chickpeas), whole grains, nuts, and unsaturated fatty acids (especially olive and canola oil) and modest amounts of wine. It may also include low or no fat varieties of dairy products.

Starting in the 1950s it was noted that people eating the Mediterranean diet, particularly on the island of Crete, had very low rates of heart disease and cancers, as well as long life expectancy. While other factors, notably exercise and strong social networks contributed, the Mediterranean diet is believed to have been the primary factor in the good health enjoyed by the region.

As modern styles of eating took hold in the area – with the rapid growth of supermarkets, convenience foods, and advertising aimed at children – health in the region deteriorated profoundly. A meteoric rise in obesity, high cholesterol, diabetes and other cardiovascular risks occurred, especially among children.

Since the 1950s, many studies have linked the traditional Mediterranean diet with striking health benefits, including reduced heart disease, diabetes, cancer, obesity, inflammation, cholesterol, and metabolic syndrome (a collection of early symptoms of heart disease and diabetes).

The Anti-Inflammatory Diet that Changed My Life

While researching the links between nutrition, inflammation and chronic disease for Greater Boston Physicians for Social Responsibility, I began to experiment with a diet based on the nutrition principles that were arising from our research. The diet I adopted, an anti-inflammatory diet, is my own rather intense application of these principles, without regard for convenience or popular acceptability.

While components of the anti-inflammatory diet have been studied, and found to have many benefits, this particular diet as a whole is untested. Thus my experience, like any anecdotal case, should be considered a personal story that may point the way forward.

That said, this diet changed my life. Starting in my mid-fifties, when health is usually going downhill, mine took a dramatic turn for the better.

Almost immediately on starting the diet, my concentration and memory – specifically my recall of events, facts and words - became sharper than at any time in my life. Rather suddenly, my struggle to integrate mountains of studies into a coherent framework for our book became almost easy. At the same time, my occasional symptoms of American malaise disappeared, including episodic insomnia, low grade anxiety and occasional bouts of mild depression.

Within weeks my chronic asthma went into complete remission. My occasional migraine headaches (including "auras" in which I would transiently lose vision) disappeared, and oddly, my tendency to become carsick vanished. Another surprise was that my typically dreadful experience of the common cold came to an end. In fact I stopped contracting colds at all, even when family members brought viral illnesses back to our home.

Once on the diet, I felt so much healthier and more energetic that I became passionately motivated to stay on it, even now after nearly 10 years of strict compliance. When I deviate from the diet, by consuming bread, chips, pastries, cheese, milk, ice cream etc., within minutes my concentration and memory backslide from the clarity I've become accustomed to. A few meals off the diet generally reactivate my asthma and migraines. In fact, I've become so adapted to fresh, unprocessed, plant-based food that commercial processed foods have become distasteful and unappealing to me. Being more repelled than tempted by rich or processed foods, I rarely depart from the diet.

I had good reason to try an anti-inflammatory diet, despite the inconvenience. Both of my parents had suffered long and tragic declines from Alzheimer's disease. So, I was extremely motivated to find a way to reduce the risks. The thousands of studies reviewed for our book gave us compelling scientific reason to believe an anti-inflammatory diet could be effective.

The anti-inflammatory diet is a Paleolithic diet, meaning that it excludes most of the foods that have entered the diets of civilized societies since about 8,000 BCE (when agriculture and animal domestication began), including especially the processed foods of the past century. Many of these "modern" foods drive inflammation in the body. Grains, for example, which entered the human diet 10,000 years ago, trigger a rapid rise in blood sugar. This leads to a cascade of metabolic effects that activate the immune system, causing insulin resistance and paving the way to diabetes and other chronic diseases. In general, our 10-million+ year old genes are poorly equipped to handle these additions to the human diet that are extremely recent in the time frame of human evolution. Thus, the anti-inflammatory diet excludes historically "novel" foods including grains, inflammatory fats (saturated fat and excess omega 6s) linked to animal domestication and grain-based over-feeding, and processed food.

The anti-inflammatory diet also limits nutrients that laboratory, animal or human studies have linked to increased immune activity. For nutrients where the evidence is incomplete and ambiguous, the diet errs on the anti-inflammatory side. This is the case for omega-6 fatty acids, which the anti-inflammatory diet reduces by using largely olive, or canola oil, (which is rich in omega-3s and relatively low in omega-6s) rather than other vegetable oils that have high levels of omega-6s. It also limits the intake of most nuts (which are high in omega-6s) except for walnuts (which are high in omega-3s).

As noted, the evidence for these dietary strategies is not clear cut. So, the anti-inflammatory diet should be acknowledged as something of an experiment. In my case at least, the experiment has been transformative.

The anti-inflammatory diet, in effect, deprives your immune system of the building blocks of key inflammatory mediators, many of which are built out of omega-6 fatty acids. No inflammatory mediators, no inflammation. If there's no active inflammation, then phlegm/mucus production, pain, blood vessel and heart disease, brain inflammation and other consequences of inflammation are markedly reduced, and many symptoms of inflammatory disease improve. This is vastly oversimplified, of course. But the general point is correct.

The importance of diet as a foundation of health underscores the importance of ensuring universal access to affordable nutritious, sustainably grown food for all. It is an intolerable injustice that tax dollars are currently used to subsidize industrial food-like substances that are making us sick on a global scale. We should be subsidizing local, sustainably grown, plant-based foods that are not only desirable, but also essential for human and planetary health.

Ultimately, the quest for healthy, sustainable food is a political battle, increasingly waged against multinational agribusiness corporations and the political establishment that serves them. These profit driven corporations are destroying nutritious food systems and replacing them with sickening industrial foods, while poisoning land, water, farmers and agricultural communities with toxic pesticides, and eliminating crop diversity with GMOs. Likewise, they are destroying forests and stealing indigenous lands around the world to create industrial farms.

Against these predators stand a multitude of compassionate individuals: Indigenous nations, farming families, fair trade advocates and consumers. Our lives will ultimately depend on winning this battle, not only for food justice, but for climate justice, economic justice, labor justice and racial justice. Working together, in a unifying struggle for people, planet and peace over profit, we are an unstoppable and inspired force. Eating an anti-inflammatory diet is one way to improve and maintain our health, so we can wage this battle for justice on the long road ahead.

References:

[i] Gikas A, Sotiropoulos A, Panagiotakos D, et al. Rising prevalence of diabetes among Greek adults: findings from two consecutive surveys in the same target population. Diabetes Res Clin Pract. 2008 Feb;79(2):325-9. Epub 2007 Oct 23.

[ii] Gikas A, Sotiropoulos A, et al. Prevalence trends for myocardial infarction and conventional risk factors among Greek adults (2002-06). QJM. 2008 Sep;101(9):705-12. Epub 2008 Jul 4. QJM. 2008 Sep;101(9):741-2.

[iii] Tzotzas T, Krassas GE. Prevalence and trends of obesity in children and adults of South Europe. Pediatr Endocrinol Rev. 2004 Aug;1 Suppl 3:448-54.

[iv] De Logeril et al. Med. diet, traditional risk factors, and the rate of cardiovascular complications after myocardial infarction: final report of the Lyon Diet Heart Study. Circulation. 1999 Feb 16;99(6):779-85.

[v] BarziF, et al. Mediterranean diet and all-causes mortality after myocardial infarction: results from the GISSIPrevenzione trial European Journal of Clinical Nutrition (2003) 57, 604–611

[vi] Estruch R, Martínez-González MA, Corella D, et al. Effects of a Mediterranean-style diet on cardiovascular risk factors: a randomized trial. Ann Intern Med. 2006 Jul 4;145(1):1-11.

[vii] Serra-Majem et al. Scientific evidence of interventions using the Mediterranean diet: a systematic review. Nutr Reviews 2006 Feb;64(2 Pt 2):S27-47.

[viii] Vincent-Baudry S. The Medi-RIVAGE study: reduction of cardiovascular disease risk factors after a 3-mo intervention with a Mediterranean-type diet or a low-fat diet. Am J Clin Nutr. 2005 Nov;82(5):964-71.

[ix] Esposito, K, et al. Effect of a Med-style diet on endothelial dysfunction and markers of vascular inflammation in the metabolic syndrome. Random. Trial. JAMA 292(2):1440-6, 2004.

[x] Vincent-Baudry S. The Medi-RIVAGE study: reduction of cardiovascular disease risk factors after a 3-mo intervention with a Mediterranean-type diet or a low-fat diet. Am J Clin Nutr. 2005 Nov;82(5):964-71.

[xi] Estruch R, Martínez-González MA, Corella D, et al. Effects of a Mediterranean-style diet on cardiovascular risk factors: a randomized trial. Ann Intern Med. 2006 Jul 4;145(1):1-11.

[xii] Serra-Majem, et al. Scientific evidence of interventions using the Mediterranean diet: a systematic review. Nutr Reviews 2006 Feb;64(2 Pt 2):S27-47.

[xiii] Vincent-Baudry S. The Medi-RIVAGE study: reduction of cardiovascular disease risk factors after a 3-mo intervention with a Mediterranean-type diet or a low-fat diet. Am J Clin Nutr. 2005 Nov;82(5):964-71.

[xiv] Estruch R, Martínez-González MA, Corella D, et al. Effects of a Mediterranean-style diet on cardiovascular risk factors: a randomized trial. Ann Intern Med. 2006 Jul 4;145(1):1-11.

[xv] Serra-Majem, et al. Scientific evidence of interventions using the Mediterranean diet: a systematic review. Nutr Reviews 2006 Feb;64(2 Pt 2):S27-47.

[xvi] Vincent-Baudry S. The Medi-RIVAGE study: reduction of cardiovascular disease risk factors after a 3-mo intervention with a Mediterranean-type diet or a low-fat diet. Am J Clin Nutr. 2005 Nov;82(5):964-71.

[xvii] Esposito, K et al. Effect of a Med-style diet on endothelial dysfunction and markers of vascular inflammation in the metabolic syndrome. Random. Trial. JAMA 292(2):1440-6, 2004.

[xviii] Shai I, Schwarzfuchs D, Henkin, et al. Weight loss with a low-carbohydrate, Mediterranean, or low-fat diet. N Engl J Med. 2008 Jul 17;359(3):229-41.

[xix] Vincent-Baudry S. The Medi-RIVAGE study: reduction of cardiovascular disease risk factors after a 3-mo intervention with a Mediterranean-type diet or a low-fat diet. Am J Clin Nutr. 2005 Nov;82(5):964-71.

[xx] Esposito, K, et al. Effect of a Med-style diet on endothelial dysfunction and markers of vascular inflammation in the metabolic syndrome. Random. Trial. JAMA 292(2):1440-6, 2004.

[xxi] Estruch R, Martínez-González MA, Corella D, et al. Effects of a Mediterranean-style diet on cardiovascular risk factors: a randomized trial. Ann Intern Med. 2006 Jul 4;145(1):1-11.

[xxii] Martínez-González MA, et al. Adherence to Mediterranean diet and risk of developing diabetes: prospective cohort study. BMJ. 2008 Jun 14;336(7657):1348-51. Epub 2008 May 29.

[xxiii] van Dam RM. Dietary patterns and risk for type 2 diabetes mellitus in U.S. men. Ann Intern Med. 2002 Feb 5;136(3):201-9.

[xxiv] Brunner EJ, Mosdøl A, Witte DR, et al. Dietary patterns and 15-y risks of major coronary events, diabetes, and mortality. Am J Clin Nutr. 2008 May;87(5):1414-21.

[xxv] Benetou V, et al. Conformity to traditional Mediterranean diet and cancer incidence: the Greek EPIC cohort. Br J Cancer. 2008 Jul 8;99(1):191-5.

[xxvi] Sofi F, Cesari F, Abbate R, Gensini GF, Casini A. Adherence to Mediterranean diet and health status: meta-analysis. BMJ. 2008 Sep 11;337.

Introduction

Can Changing What You Eat Really Change Your Life?
My Story: How I lost 60 pounds in six months.

In developing and following the Vitality Anti-Inflammatory Diet, I lost all the baby weight I gained while pregnant, and then lost an additional 20 pounds in six months without going to the gym and without being hungry. I still have a hard time believing the diet worked, and I'm still losing weight. I was 145 pounds and a size 12 when I became pregnant in March of 2013. I gained 40 pounds in the nine months before my son was born, topping out at 185. I'm now a size 4 and 20 pounds lighter than before I got pregnant! People don't even recognize me. At a charity event, I sat next to a colleague of my husband who hadn't seen me in six months and when I said hello, she didn't recognize me. I said, "It's me, Sarah, remember?" and she said, "Oh! You look different." I said, "Yes, I look skinny." and she said, "I didn't want to be rude but you were much bigger before." I even had someone call me tiny recently.

I'm writing this book to help those kindred spirits who are also trying to lose weight and reclaim their health. I feel so fortunate to have finally found something easy that works!

I struggled for years – more than a decade – trying to lose weight with every possible combination of exercise and diet and supplements and never lost more than 10 pounds. It was like the weight was never coming off! I am a problem solver by nature and I poured through the research online, looking at the science behind why people gain and lose weight. Everywhere I looked the advice was to cut calories, which, as I later discovered, is very difficult and usually counterproductive. I decided that based on my height of 5'5" I had to cut my calories to 1,200 – 1,500 per day to even begin to lose weight. I also believed that I would have to go to the gym almost every day and alternate between cardiovascular (elliptical machine, etc.) and weight lifting.

I kept a log of everything I ate every day. This was a lot of work and removed the joy from eating, but I was committed to losing weight and so I kept a calorie log for over a year. I succeeded in keeping my calorie intake below 1,500 calories per day and exercised at least five days a week. I hired a personal trainer to make sure I was alternating exercises efficiently. And after all that I still didn't lose more than a pound or two. It was incredibly disheartening. I started to consider reducing the food I was eating to 500 calories per day because I saw a video of a woman who lost weight with a tube up her nose that fed her only 500 calories per day. This is the so-called K-E Diet which costs $1,500 for the 10-day plan, seems yucky, extreme, dangerous, and totally unworkable over the long term. I didn't try extreme calorie restriction because I knew it would make me miserable and that it would probably slow my metabolism and make it even harder to lose weight in the future. But I considered it. I really do understand how frustrating weight loss can be.

This book offers a path to health and weight loss that doesn't include calorie cutting. Why? Because calorie restriction slows your metabolism. And being hungry is very unpleasant.

What is Metabolism?

When people talk about metabolism they're referring to the biochemical processes occurring within any living organism - humans and animals - to maintain life. These biochemical processes allow us to grow, reproduce, repair damage, and respond to our environment. In simple terms, our body weight is a result of the amount of energy we release into our bodies minus the amount of energy our bodies use. The excess energy is stored as fat. It is a common belief that slim people have a "high metabolism" while overweight/obese people have a "low metabolism". However, this is overstated because what is really affecting the amount of fat stored in your body is the amount of inflammatory food you eat.

Severely restricting your caloric intake will make you miserable and your metabolism will bottom out. When you are following a very-low-calorie eating plan, your metabolism slows down as a protective mechanism. Your basal metabolic rate - the amount of energy used when you're resting for breathing, circulation, digestion and so on, accounts for up to 75 percent of the calories your body uses each day. Your body will always prioritize completing these activities, because they are essential for life. So if there are very few calories available because you are starving yourself, your metabolism will slow way down so that essential functions continue. If that happens, it becomes far more difficult to achieve weight loss. In contrast to calorie cutting, you will lose weight eating the Vitality Diet no matter regardless of your basic metabolism.

Got it? *Great!* Back to my story.

I started to believe that maybe my body wanted to be a certain weight and that I would never be able to lose the weight no matter how much I exercised. I thought maybe if I was a runner I would lose the weight. However, I can't run because I have a condition called "runner's itch" or *cholinergic urticaria*. Thousands of people suffer from it. When I run, after about 5 minutes I start to feel a tingling in my legs that rapidly develops into an insanely painful itch that's so bad you want to start crying and scratch the skin right off your legs.

I also tried meal replacement protein shakes with no luck. I even tried things that I knew in my heart wouldn't work, like expensive pills you find at GNC, i.e. Hydroxycut and Total Lean. I figured these pills must work for some people. But I was fooling myself. And the pills made me feel jittery and would often make my stomach hurt. I didn't feel good about not knowing what was in each pill - many of which are made in other countries in factories with little production oversight. I had a nagging feeling that they could be filled with nothing, or worse, with poison, and I wouldn't know. Unlike regular food or drugs, supplements aren't regulated closely by the U.S. Food and Drug Administration (FDA). Although dietary supplement manufacturers must register their facilities with the FDA, they are not required to get FDA approval before producing or selling dietary supplements. Manufacturers and distributors are supposed to make sure that all claims and information on the product label and in other labeling are truthful and not misleading, but I'm pretty sure no one is checking out each and every stupendous claim.

Finally, a very energetic and skinny 60+ year old medical doctor named Jill Stein told me about the anti-inflammatory diet. She said that she had started to suffer from all the "normal" aging diseases like weight gain, ovarian cysts, high blood pressure, a foggy mind, declining energy, and more. Close members of her family suffered from Alzheimer's disease and she believed that if she didn't take drastic action that would be her fate as well. Being a Harvard trained medical doctor, she poured through the published medical research searching for ways to cure and prevent Alzheimer's and she discovered the literature on inflammation as a root cause of disease in our bodies.

Dr. Stein told me that she made the commitment to eating only anti-inflammatory foods and not only did she lose weight, but she experienced a much more vital immune system, mental function, and psychological condition. All the "normal" old age conditions that she had been suffering from disappeared, and she started to have the clarity of mind of her youth. I listened to her, but I didn't take immediate action. It just seemed too good to be true.

Then I got pregnant. I was extremely happy about having a baby! And, like many women, I was terrified of gaining too much weight and then never being able to lose it, which would set me even further back from my goal. Now that I was pregnant, I couldn't keep up the calorie restriction and the daily hour at the gym. I had read that you can have a healthy baby and still only gain 25 pounds, so I made a commitment to myself and my baby to eat healthy foods and walk as much as possible. And for the most part I did eat healthy – and you know if you've been pregnant - the only thing you really want to eat is carbs. Pizza, pasta, macaroni and cheese never looked better and I developed a strong aversion to the greens and the salads I used to eat daily. I walked at least an hour every day, so much so that my doctor told me to stop walking because the baby was getting too big. (To be clear: It's not certain that exercising while pregnant produces a bigger baby).

Well, I blew past 25 pounds around month five and gained 40 pounds. Here's an unaltered picture of me right before my son was born.

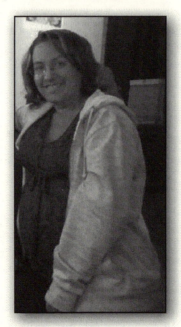

After the birth, I figured it was lose the weight now or never. Either I give up and remain heavy for the rest of my life or try one last thing, the anti-inflammatory diet. I decided to give it a try, because I wanted my son to feel proud of me and I wanted to feel better about myself. With a new baby at home, it was very tough to get back to the gym. So, I looked at a one-page flyer given to me by Dr. Stein that listed the foods with anti-inflammatory properties and I started to cook using only those ingredients. It was surprisingly easy and I developed several tasty recipes by varying the base or main ingredient and toppings.

Today is the First Day of the Rest of Your Life.
What I'm offering here is a total life change for the better. The Vitality Diet is a permanent weight loss solution and what's even better is that you will be healthy. Really healthy. You won't just look better, you'll feel better. And, compared to the pain of failure, the hours at the gym, and the misery of disease; the life style changes listed here are easy. After a month or two you won't even have to think about it anymore. You will wake up each day feeling refreshed with a clear mind and a healthy, thinner body. You will feel proud of yourself for being a responsible adult and making the lifestyle changes necessary to maintain a healthy weight. No one can stop you or hold you back. This is your destiny.

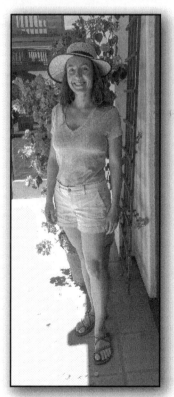

Part 1: Understanding the Science

CHAPTER 1
What is Inflammation?

The word inflammation comes from Latin *inflammo*, meaning, "I set alight," or "I ignite." Inflammation is more than heat and redness, it is the body's attempt to protect itself by removing harmful stimuli, including damaged cells, ingested toxins, irritants, or pathogens, and begin the healing process. When something harmful or irritating affects a part of our body, like when you eat processed foods, inflammation is the biological response to try to remove it. The signs and symptoms of inflammation, specifically acute inflammation, show that the body is trying to heal itself.

Inflammation is deeply linked to some of our society's most common chronic illnesses a deadly diseases. Chronic inflammation can cause some cancers, rheumatoid arthritis, atherosclerosis, periodontitis, and hay fever. Asthma, for example, is often caused by inflammation of the airways. Ulcers are a classic example of how inflammation can damage an organ, creating a sore in the lining of the stomach. Tuberculosis is not directly caused by inflammation, but it is spurred by it, as is sinusitis. Some of the most common chronic diseases like hepatitis, Crohn's disease, and arthritis are all caused by inflammation.

But where does inflammation come from? Some inflammation is caused by long-term stress on the body, however most of the inflammation we experience comes from the food we eat. The food we put into our bodies has a huge effect on the level of inflammation and how it affects us. Even in its mildest forms, inflammation caused by food can interrupt the metabolism and make it impossible for the body to utilize calories correctly, causing you to gain weight. In its most serious forms, inflammation can cause widespread havoc in the body, attacking the digestive, circulatory, skeletal, and even nervous systems.

If you are having trouble losing weight and feel constantly "under the weather," inflammation is probably playing a significant role in your poor health. A blood test looking for C-reactive proteins can reveal hidden inflammation. Hidden inflammation takes a toll on the body, which often has the most serious long-term effects, since it is "hidden" and therefore allowed to lie dormant for years before it starts to become a serious noticeable problem.

CHAPTER 2
What Inflammation Looks Like

Most people do not notice inflammation in their daily lives unless they already have a disease or condition that is caused by, or which causes, increased levels of inflammation. For example, if you have sprained your ankle, you know what inflammation, in one of its forms, looks and feels like. The body sends fluids like blood to the sprain to help cushion and heal it, swelling the area. This is natural, expected, and what we want to happen when we have an injury.

The same thing happens when you have a sore throat. An infection invades the body. To combat the infection, the body becomes inflamed. You get a fever and your throat feels hot and scratchy. Again, this is natural, expected, and desired. In short, inflammation is the body's response to an injury or to something unwanted in its system.

What isn't natural, expected, or desired, however, is the kind of inflammation that occurs in reaction to the food we eat. Inflammation is a defense mechanism, and an effective one, but when the body is chronically inflamed, you will be sick. It's like an immune system wildfire. Not only does the fire clear out the bad things, it kills the good things, too.

CHAPTER 3
Why Inflammation Makes You Fat

Just like your body sends fluid to the site of a sprain, it will send fluid all over your body when you eat a high-inflammation diet. This means you retain above normal amounts of fluid, feel bloated, and have trouble losing weight in the long term, so long as you keep feeding the fire of inflammation.

Inflammation is especially destructive to your digestive tract, which is why stomach ulcers are so common. Inflammation also directly disrupts your body's ability to correctly process the food it eats (even the good foods). Why? Because your body behaves as if it is in crisis mode. It wants to retain as many calories as possible in order to feed itself as it fights this on-going battle. Unfortunately, the calories that are getting stored are feeding the inflammation.

A little more than half of the adults in the United States are overweight. Statistics show that an incredible 65 percent of the U.S. population is considered to be "overweight" or "obese." If you suffer from inflammation, this forces your adrenal glands to secrete hormones that destabilize your insulin and blood sugar levels. The body's metabolism breaks down and the body stops burning fat. Rather than making use of the food you eat, your body stores it, making you feel bloated and tired. You can't use the energy you gain from food and you can't burn the leftover fat, increasing your weight gain dramatically. Toxins accumulate and you feel awful.

It is interesting to note that the body doesn't add more fat cells after puberty. Our already present fat cells expand and grow as we add on weight. Swollen fat cells can leak into the surrounding tissue, leading to inflammation. Macrophages, soldiers of the immune system, are deployed to clean up this leakage. They release an inflammatory chemical during the process, one that only adds fuel to the fire.

Leptin is a hormone present in everyone. Its primary function is to maintain the appropriate weight level of the body. We've all seen those rare people that can eat anything and everything and never put on an ounce. Their leptin is high functioning, able to stave off the effects of immense overeating. It does this by boosting their metabolism and using other controls, such as suppressing the appetite, to maintain a healthy ratio. However, if the leptin response encounters an inflammatory response, it will be rendered ineffective. No longer will leptin control appetite or alter your metabolism. This leaves your body struggling to maintain a normal weight as it becomes a victim of inflammation.

You can, however, reverse leptin resistance. Leptin interference can be corrected and, as a result, you will have help maintaining a healthy weight. Losing weight can substantially increase the efficiency of leptin, and following a healthy eating plan can assure your success in normalizing your leptin levels.

CHAPTER 4
Why Inflammation Makes You Sick

Inflammation itself can make you sick. Just like holding your hand over a flame, when you maintain a constant state of inflammation, you are going to suffer. But there is also a deeper connection between experiencing inflammation and feeling sick. Many of the foods that cause this inflammation in humans are foods to which humans are allergic or intolerant.

Just like any other animal, there are some things we are not supposed to eat. Unlike animals, however, we do not always listen to our bodies and we eat those 'foods' anyway. While the general allergic response is not as severe as it is for those who have a peanut allergy or a severe gluten intolerance, it does exist. Besides making you feel down and distracting your immune system from other, perhaps more pressing issues, it causes long-term inflammation. Most people have a mild intolerance for wheat and dairy, for example, but continue to eat them, usually because they are not aware of their own mild intolerance. The effects of eating a slice of bread or drinking a glass of milk are almost always long-term and cumulative, not short term and urgent. Since we don't immediately feel the need to rush to the emergency room, we don't usually recognize that we are harming ourselves.

Avoiding inflammatory foods and increasing consumption of anti-inflammatory foods and activities like exercise can help you get out of the fat and sick cycle.

Inflammation is how the body responds to illness or infection. Inflammation is at its most basic an immune function. It's a protective response in reaction to things the body sees as potential sources of danger to its (your) survival. This process is a complex mechanism of immune cells combined with clotting proteins and signaling molecules. And, most importantly, your body's immune response "learns" and changes throughout your life.

Your immune system works nonstop around the clock, protecting your body, from infection. Infection, often confused with inflammation, is merely the invasion of pathogens in your body. Inflammation is the body's response to what it considers a threat to health. Your immune system is almost entirely invisible in the execution of its duties. In fact, you never know that it's working, until it stops working or has a proverbial hiccup.

For example, getting a simple cut can allow bacteria into your body. The pathogens travel easily through your first layer of protection - your skin - into your body and bloodstream. More often than not, your body can respond accordingly and your immune system, essentially, destroys every possible hazard to your body with ease and efficiency. This allows your skin to heal and repair itself, restoring your protective layer from further potential pathogenic infiltration.

However, sometimes the immune system misses something. Everyone has experienced that one cut that becomes reddened and inflamed, pus building-up into something unpleasant. The inflammation is gross to look at, but it's natural. If something does get through, that pus, that inflammation, is the second layer of protection your body deploys. Its "yell" is in the form of a class of biochemicals called cytokines, which beckon to other white blood cells to come to the point of infection and surround the enemy.

Most often all this goes unnoticed because the first few white blood cells engulf and digest the invaders. If they're not able to kill the invaders, more and more white blood cells congregate at the site, trapping the pathogens in the center. This build up is blob of pus under the skin.

For another example, you might inhale a cold germ, but your body can and will fight it off most of the time. You most likely get over those little health problems because your immune system is resilient and amazing. In fact, if it weren't for our immune system we wouldn't be able to eat without killing ourselves. Our food has germs all over it, thousands upon thousands of them. Our saliva and stomach acid are usually capable of neutralizing these germs on contact and keeping us safe. If a dangerous germ does get through and penetrate those protective layers, our immune system goes into overdrive, giving us the tell-tale symptoms of food poisoning. While the accompanying diarrhea and/or vomiting is unappealing, it is almost always necessary.

But, there are downsides to our wonderful immune system.

Food allergies are a growing epidemic. The latest numbers show nearly 15 million people in the United States suffer from food allergies. What's most concerning is that

1 in 13 children are reported to suffer from food allergies. Sadly, not only are food allergies potentially life threatening, but its common knowledge that they are intrinsically tied to weight issues as well as chronic inflammation.

A food allergy, superficially, is identical to other kinds of immune responses. For some reason, the immune system gets "wacky" and decides to treat certain substances as dangerous. The histamine reaction and the subsequent inflammation come along for the ride. These allergies, while often discovered during childhood, can develop at any time. You could develop an allergy to foods you have enjoyed for years, then all of a sudden the itchy, burning sensations begin when you eat them. Those simple food proteins are viewed as dangerous by immune cells and are sought out and marked for destruction.

If you suffer from any of the following symptoms, you will see remarkable benefits after even just one week of eating anti-inflammatory foods. Chronic fatigue, depression, craving for breads and sugars, extreme mood swings, hypoglycemia, excessive mucus in your throat, nose, and lungs, chronic fungal infections of the skin (jock itch, athlete's foot) or vaginal/oral thrush, diarrhea, urinary tract and acute kidney infections, cystitis, prostatitis, short-term memory loss, or feeling bloated or gassy after eating. In addition, lymphatic swelling, difficult PMS, night sweats, chest and joint pain, memory loss, loss of coordination, blurred vision, arthritis, intense, random headaches, intermittent vertigo, insomnia, sneezing fits, and increased food allergies are also signs that you could benefit from a diet rich in anti-inflammatory foods. Your body could be suffering from an overload and abundance of toxins that is making you sick.

Being sick, essentially, is when your body is running at less than optimal level. You can't perform at your usual level of activity and things just generally slow down internally. Of course, there are multiple sources of "getting sick". Just a few examples are:

- **Mechanical damage** – Quite visible, sometimes you just have a physical problem. You might break a bone, or tear a ligament. This is, basically, making you sick. You can't perform up to your personal standards and your abilities are inhibited.
- **Vitamin or mineral deficiency** – Not getting the recommended daily intake of various vitamins can have a huge impact on your health. Vitamin D, A, C, are all essential just to maintain normal bodily functions. Without them, you risk a multitude of disease and lower than anticipated capacities for health.

- **Organ degradation** – An organ can be weakened by one or more factors. Eating too much bad cholesterol can lead to heart disease, degrading your heart function and stifling its ability to suffocation. This greatly limits its capabilities as a central organ, one necessary for survival. Your liver can be damaged through various means or simply old fashioned bad luck; however ingesting large amounts of alcohol could expedite a damaging process. Your lungs can also suffer from inhalation of foreign bodies and smoke, damaging their lining and reducing their functional capacity. Some of these forms of organ degradation are avoidable, but not all.
- **Genetic disease** – We're all built of DNA, a series of codes and proteins. Genetic disease, however, is a coding error that gets implanted into the DNA sequence. Often, these errors produce issues with protein production that can drastically impact your body at a cellular level. Sickle-cell disease and cystic fibrosis are examples of a genetic disease/disorder, present at birth.
- **Cancer** – Every so often, a cell mutates. A malfunction in the nucleus causes it not to recognize those cells around it. It starts to multiply, and surround itself with cells and continues to regenerate. The cells it produces are just as faulty as the original and the cancer grows. This reaction can be spontaneous without an outside factor, but it can also be due to outside factors such as sunlight exposure (that can lead to melanoma) or the inhalation of smoke that can lead to lung cancer.

Inflammation, therefore, is a way that your body can keep you healthy. It's like a military reaction to an invasion. The troops are dispatched, the reserves called up, and a full attack is launched until the threat is neutralized. Those troops, our white blood cells, are our line of defense against pathogenic invasion.

One issue with this, of course, is that sometimes our white blood cells are called up too often, and too aggressively. They start to lose focus and can't tell good cells from bad. Stressing our system with toxic food can lead to an always alert immune system, one that seeks to neutralize first and ask questions later. This can lead to chronic inflammation where the body's normal, healthy cells are misidentified and attacked. This, in itself, can lead to recurrent, chronic problems such as heart disease or Crohn's disease. These friendly fire attacks can occur in tissues at almost any location in the body and drain all of your reserve energy.

Chronically inflamed bodies don't have the ability to do anything else but keep fighting off real and unreal invaders. There's no energy left for the work of digestion of the food you're currently eating and your body starts to get lazy, storing food as fat to deal with later. It doesn't have the time or resources to do anything else. Eventually, the buildup keeps expanding and you get weaker and weaker. You can't produce the energy necessary to deal with the excessive fat and you can't heal the havoc produced by your overactive immune system.

What is pain?

Pain is the tell-tale sign of injury, of inflammation. Pain is your body's way of warning you that by moving, you are doing damage. Chronic pain can be thought of as a train crossing warning light. If you don't move off the tracks, you're eventually going to get slammed with something really unpleasant. You'll notice the pain of inflammation before you notice anything else. You might see redness with a surface injury, but you won't truly notice it until the throbbing/burning begins. If it becomes intense, you'll likely take a pain pill or visit the doctor for some sort of momentary relief.

However, like those over-the-counter forms of relief, most medications are simply a temporary fix. Most doctors don't care to offer up an explanation of what inflammation is, if they even understand it themselves. Their major intent when treating inflammation, or pain of any kind, is to provide relief. If that is done, then they consider their job complete. This well-intentioned goal doesn't really help you in the long run. An investigative attempt at identifying the source of your inflammatory pain is not only costly, but most doctors will most likely believe it to be unnecessary. So, the drugs they prescribe, while seemingly effective, are masking an underlying problem.

Don't let yourself fall into that trap of being complacent with temporary removal of pain. You might feel fine, but you could also be sick. Inflammation, like cancer, is a quiet, lurking disease. One that you don't know you have until it storms to the forefront and makes itself known. By then, it may be too late because your body will be too exhausted to heal itself. If you have silent inflammation, you're sick.

You have to be aware, always, of how your body works. You need to recognize those key symptoms of inflammation and stop them before your body overreacts. If your body goes into a meltdown, it will be much harder to pick yourself back up. If you catch it early enough, you can ease into a routine of eating health-affirming, anti-inflammatory foods. However, if things are already on a downhill tragectory, you can still jump in with drastic changes to your diet now to salvage your health and your future.

If you've already been diagnosed with chronic, especially destructive diseases such as cancer or Alzheimer's, quick action is necessary. Immediate action. Even the mainstream medical community has started to notice the immediate effects that anti-inflammatory foods can have on general well-being as well as fighting disease.

Luckily, inflammation is reversible. If you already have a healthy body weight and active lifestyle, you might not be in as much danger. But, if you eat poorly and are less active than you should be, or are suffering from a chronic disease, you need to take immediate action and correct your course to prevent falling even further into the inflammation trap. You need to motivate yourself to become more active, and eat healthier. The anti-inflammatory diet is a way to achieve health, not only by reducing the damaging food that you intake, but also by counteracting any present inflammation. No matter what the illness, what the disease, there is great potential to heal yourself with food.

CHAPTER 5
Candida Yeast and Other Yeast Infections

If you ask most people what they think about yeast, they will probably tell you that it's used in baking. But there is yeast that occurs naturally in our environment (that's how sourdough bread was first made), and not all of that yeast is good. Some yeast can help promote good bacteria growth, but bad yeast can promote the growth of bad bacteria.

Candida Albicans
This is the most common kind of yeast in the world and is very different from the kind of yeast that bakers use in bread. It can grow and multiply in the body, living in our bloodstream and in our organs, causing rampant inflammation and making it difficult for the body to function properly. If you often feel tired or are chronically fatigued, this kind of yeast could be a big part of that problem.

How does it survive? Like all yeast, it lives on sugar, and because most Westerners eat a very high-sugar diet (even if they do not realize they are doing it), Candida albicans has plenty of fuel to grow inside the body, sapping you of essential nutrients. It's like having a giant tapeworm throughout your entire body that absorbs all of the energy that you should be using.

Foods that Feed the Yeast Beast
You don't have to be constantly eating candy in order for the bad yeast inside your body to be happily fed. In fact, you can cut all traditional sources of sugar, like candy, cake, and cookies, out of your diet, and you will still be getting plenty of sugar to feed

the yeast. Where does it come from? Mostly from processed foods like white bread, dairy, and junk food.

This yeast does not need much time to become the dominant flora in your gut, which means your immune system could be quickly impacted. A poor diet feeds this yeast, while a healthy one can starve it out. Blood tests check for IgG, IgA, and IgM Candida antibodies in your blood, and can be performed at most any lab.

CHAPTER 6

Before, We Had Little to Eat: An Evolutionary Explanation behind Our Cravings for Sugar and Fat

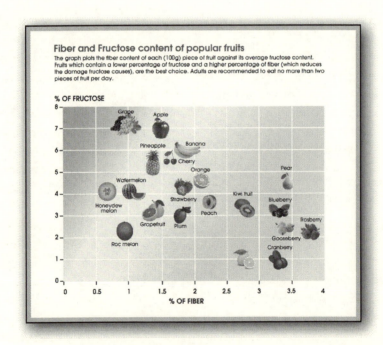

There's an evolutionary reason why when you see a McDonald's commercial that those fries *do* look good to eat. Or you feel yourself wanting a cookie or a donut - something sugary or full of fat - as soon as possible. Whether you're sitting in an office, ten feet from the box of donuts your boss just dropped off, or at home, just a few steps away from a snack cupboard full of chips or crackers, you may find your willpower lacking.

But why does this happen? Why do we suddenly get an overwhelming craving for anything that contains sugar or fat? Unfortunately, this is not just a learned response. It's not just from those childhood experiences when Mom or Dad was too tired to cook so they took you to your favorite fast food restaurant. It's in our DNA.

Our primate ancestors subsisted on a high sugar and fat diet. Primates seek out ripe fruit because, the riper the fruit, the higher the sugar content, and the more energy obtained from it. The same goes for fatty foods - fat was rare, sugar was rare - the fat and sugar found kept individuals alive. Because fat and sugar were so rare, our genetic ancestors became hyper efficient at turning sugar into fat. Those evolutionary biological traits and the impulse to seek out sugar and fat still exist, but unlike in our Cro-Magnon days, fatty and sugary foods are now extremely easy to find.

1,000 years ago cavemen and cavewomen weren't munching a donut every time they got a craving, but dining on donuts is definitely a possibility for us. Even the positive emotions that we feel (usually only initially) when eating junk food can be linked back to these ancestors, who surely would celebrate when a hunting or gathering party brought back a huge basket of sweet fruit. In the past, we needed these calories to survive. We still need calories, but only if we eat the same kinds of sugar and fats that our ancestors ate. That means fruits, vegetables, and healthy protein like nuts. Not donuts, fries, and cookies.

You already know how addictive sugar can be. Most people, when they cut sugar out of their lives, report serious withdrawal symptoms, ranging from headaches, irritability, and even nausea. Though we don't think of sugar as a drug, it definitely can be. It's addictive and dangerous, especially for those with blood sugar issues, heart problems, or obesity. But our attachment to sugar is not just physical, it is also deeply emotional, which can make it even more difficult to kick the habit.

Think about every birthday party you have ever attended. What's the centerpiece of food at the party? Probably a birthday cake (or something like cake, if the child doesn't like cake). Almost every holiday (especially the big ones like Hanukkah, Christmas, Valentine's Day, and Halloween) is deeply connected to candy and baked goods. You have been trained to associate sugar with positive feelings, which can teach your brain to release those "feel-good" hormones when you eat sugar. Just think about how chocolate is marketed with every brand trying to make you think of happiness. Hershey's even has a line of chocolates called "Bliss."

Because fewer and fewer people are making real, powerful connections with others, as technology continues to dominate our lives, more and more people are craving that false happiness and satisfaction that sugar temporarily provides. It's a temporary fix for a growing problem, and more people are self-medicating with sugar than ever before. It's time to stop this toxic cycle.

If you want to lose weight and be healthy, you MUST stop eating sugar. Fat is not the problem. Think about this. Fat makes up a smaller portion of the American diet than it did 20 years ago but the number of people who are obese has grown. The average American eats more than 77 pounds of sugar a year. That equals 22 additional teaspoons of added sugar per day! We weren't meant to eat so much sugar. From the beginning of humankind, our bodies have not developed the ability to digest large amounts of added sugar. Only 600 years ago we weren't eating any added sugar in our diet. In 1900, 5 percent of adults worldwide had high blood pressure. Now one-third of adults do. In 1980 153 million people had diabetes, and now 347 million people suffer from diabetes.

If you eat too much sugar in the form of candy and soda, your liver will break down the fructose and make fats called triglycerides. Some of the fat stays in your liver, which is bad, but the majority of the triglycerides get pumped into your bloodstream. Too much exposure and your blood pressure increases and your tissues become progressively more resistant to insulin. Your pancreas responds by pouring out more insulin to make up for the resistance until metabolic syndrome kicks in and you are sapped of your energy. This is a sad statistic, but a third of American adults meet the criteria for metabolic syndrome set by the National Institutes of Health. University of California, San Francisco endocrinologist Robert Lustig says, "Sugar is a poison by itself when consumed in high doses."

Many anti-inflammatory recipes use stevia to provide a natural sweetness and replace refined sugar. Stevia scores "0" on the glycemic index. When stevia leaves are dried, the compounds stevioside and rebaudioside are extracted to give stevia its sweetness, which is about 300 times sweeter than sugar. These resulting compounds can be dried into powder or used in liquid form; either way, they are usually augmented with fillers, since the pure extract is so sweet the amounts used would be infinitesimal.

Stevia is available in many forms, including pure liquid, pure powder and both with added ingredients. I prefer liquid stevia as the dropper makes it easy to measure, but I use the powdered form as well. There are also one-for-one stevia-based sweeteners on the market that allow you to measure one cup of the mixture for one cup of sugar, but these always contain bulking agents, so stay away from them. You'll find pure stevia liquid in purified water, glycerin, or food grade alcohol. While the alcohol helps to preserve stevia longer, it's not suitable for those of us on the anti-inflammatory diet. The powder in its pure form is extremely potent, so it's often mixed with fillers such as cellulose or maltodextrin. You don't want to be eating these fillers, so use pure stevia.

When converting recipes to stevia instead of sugar, note that the weight of ingredients in your recipe will change. For example, if your recipe called for 2 cups of sugar and you replace the sugar with 2 teaspoons of stevia liquid, your recipe will be lacking a significant volume of ingredients. Different brands of stevia have different conversion rates, so see manufacturer's suggestions for conversions. Ground whole leaf stevia has a grassy, "green" flavor which doesn't disappear as easily in baked goods. Always add less stevia and add more gradually, tasting as you go - too much stevia has an overpowering, bitter, "soapy" flavor. Try different brands and different forms (powder, liquid, etc) to see which one you like best.

CHAPTER 7
Gardening Your Gut: Clearing the Field and Planting What You Want

Our gut is home to approximately 100,000,000,000,000 (100 trillion) microorganisms, a figure that sounds completely incomprehensible. A compromised gut, one that has an imbalance of good and bad bacteria, is one that is struggling to cope with a barrage of food irritants. Consider it a stomach under siege that is acting as a sponge for fat. If you want to lose fat and start shedding those unwanted pounds, you'll have to reduce inflammation caused by food irritants and clean your gut. That is the one and only way to rebuild your health. So, how do you going about fixing your digestive tract? Well, by clearing the field and planting what you want.

Here's what I mean. Don't think of yourself as a single individual. Instead, think of yourself as an ecosystem comprised of thousands of different creatures living together on one planet - your body. In an ecosystem, every living thing down to the smallest organism has a role. It's a working, functional community. We are not single organisms. We are a community. Our health is entirely dependent on other living creatures, even if we can't see them. Most of the time we don't even know that they're there.

Think about this, your gut contains 10 times more bacteria than all the cells in your entire body combined. Keep in mind that there are over 400 known different bacterial species that have been found in the human digestive tract. We're more bacterial than human!

When a baby is born, they're exceptionally vulnerable to sickness and infection because they haven't yet formed a cohesive ecological partnership in their body. They get help from their mother as she passes along part of her own "ecosystem" when the child passes through her birth canal and later in her breast milk. If you're a woman and plan on conceiving a child, it would not only be beneficial to you, but to your unborn offspring to get healthy and create a healthier place for that baby to grow. Remember breastfeeding is best!

New research has shown you can control what type of bacteria is present in your body. You must take active measures to control what type of organisms live in your digestive tract because, some bacteria are beneficial, while some are horrible. Concerning weight loss or gain, do you want the kind of bacteria that can help you, or hinder you, when it comes to maintaining or achieving your goal? Do you want the bacteria that works like a personal trainer and helps make you better food choices, or do you want the kind that metaphorically sits around and plays video games all day and eats pizza? If bacteria were a person, would you want it to be your friend? Of course, you do!

Installing a safety net of good bacteria in your body sets you up for making good food choices necessary for a healthy life. You need that built-in advantage if you're going to succeed in your weight loss goals. These good bacteria can reproduce and multiply, making you healthier and healthier as time passes. By eating the healthy food they thrive on, the good bacteria will outgrow the bad bacteria and help restore your digestion to a fully optimal state. This will, in turn, allow for the distribution of nutrients and rebalancing of your gut. In addition to eating anti-inflammatory foods, a great way to jumpstart your switch is to buy probiotics. When shopping for your best solution, look for the ones offering huge numbers of live organisms. Search out and locate those containing between 10-40 billion live organisms per dosage/serving. These are the ones that are most beneficial to your gut. Also, try to locate those containing Lactobacillus and Bifidobacteria. These probiotic additions can help out dramatically, but remember that they are not the "one step" solution that you might really want. They are aids and not miracles. You need to change your eating habits for the transition to really work.

Now, to really get this party started, you'll need to go for the greens. Vegetables, particularly greens, should be your go-to way of filling up. Chlorophyll in fresh greens can help heal your gut and provide the necessary nutrients to get your health and weight in line. The added benefits of the included fiber help as well, facilitating better digestive function. They work like a plumber. They can relieve constipation and clear out all the gunk that is stopping up your pipes. Things can get to moving again, and move faster. This is an essential part of building a clean, healthy body and belly. You'll lose weight and feel better by simply making greens an ever present part of your dietary intake. It's a win-win situation and your healthy body will thank you for it.

CHAPTER 8
How to Listen to Your Body

When it comes to eating, the most important thing you can do is listen to your body. You can learn to do this over time, developing this important skill and refining it. Whenever you start to get hungry, whenever that craving strikes, take this small step. It's important and something that you can learn and develop over time, but nevertheless it is essential. Ask yourself, ask your body, what it wants to eat. Clear your mind of all distractions and pause, focusing on that question. What will make you, and your body, feel the best?

You might visualize something healthy or at least acceptable. Almonds or tomato juice might be more than adequate. But, sometimes your body will go to the other end of the spectrum. Especially at the beginning of your diet transition, your body will want and crave the unhealthiest foods. Don't let that bother you. It will take time to train yourself to crave other things.

If you are craving something dramatically unhealthy, for instance, pizza, eat a handful of almonds to curb it or at least take the edge off. Then take a moment to think and determine what it is that you're craving about pizza, what is it your body is longing for? Is it the sugar in the bread? Is it the cheese? Or perhaps is it the nutrients in the sauce? Try to pinpoint exactly what it is your body is telling you that it needs. Think about each component of the food separately and see how your body reacts. If you were to just eat the crust, does that seem to you like it would taste good? Would it satisfy you? What about if you just ate a spoonful of salty and warm pizza sauce? Or ate simply melted cheese? Could you get rid of the other ingredients and still satisfy the craving you're feeling?

Is it the chewiness and mouth feel of the pizza you really want? What if you imagine yourself engaging in some other stress reducing physical activity, would this craving be reduced? Does eating pizza remind you of happy times relaxing with your mother watching a favorite movie? Often, we crave food to fill emotional needs as well as physical ones, and that's okay to have the craving, but we can still enjoy those memories without eating foods that hurt ourselves physically. What other ways can you fill your emotional need for love and closeness to other people?

You will not be able to lose weight and keep it off until you are able listen to and understand your body in this way. This is especially true because the modern food manufacturing industry has armies of "food designer" scientists combining salt, fat, sugar and chemicals together in powerful ways to manipulate the eating behavior of consumers.

You have to remember that your body is a system, a machine that is almost perfect in nature. You must listen to it rather than fight it. If you listen closely and follow its cues, you can not only lose weight, but you can overcome bad habits. There is a possibility that you have bacteria in your digestive track that loves sugar or the destructive chemicals in fast food. It was always previously thought, or assumed, that our bodies, our digestive tracts, simply lived off whatever nutrients we supplied. However, has it ever bothered you that some people crave other foods, healthier foods, and seem to truly enjoy them while you have to basically force down "health food"? Have you ever wondered why a coworker seems to enjoy salads that appear to be tasteless and bland?

Well, there's an answer for that.

Scientists from UC San Francisco, Arizona State University and University of New Mexico have proven that it is the microbes inside every one of us that influence how we eat, and our cravings. It may be difficult to think about yourself this way, but you are NOT the one that wants a particular food. It is the bacteria living in our bodies – which outnumber our own cells 100 to 1 – demanding we eat food with the particular nutrients. They are looking for what they thrive and grow on, manipulating our system to respond accordingly.

You may be wondering how these tiny microbes can control your eating behavior. The truth is, our bodies and the systems contained within, are all connected and function as a single unit for the most part. They're designed so that our gut is linked to our immune system, the endocrine system and the nervous system. Microbes in the digestive tract release signaling molecules, and those signals influence our thoughts and behavior due to this linkage. But, now that you're aware of these manipulations, you can intervene. It is even possible to destroy the unhealthy microbes that are making you sick and miserable due to their untoward influence. Think of it, in a way, like gardening. You can take control and remove the invasive creatures, and strengthen the soil (your body) and make it more fertile so that the healthy items can grow and flourish.

There is an unseen power struggle going on in your body. Your body might desire unhealthy, low nutrient food items. If that is the case, then you know which bacteria is winning the battle for your health. However, you can eliminate their food source and starve them out of existence. If you remove the sugars, and the harmful chemicals, they will have no means by which to survive. If you do this, good bacteria can begin to take over that now vacant real estate. These changes can make a dramatic impact in as little as 24 hours!

Simply altering your diet can change the microbiome of your gut drastically. However, nothing wants to die. The bad bacteria aren't going to go away quietly. For the first few days of a healthy, new diet, these lingering bacteria will scream and plead for you to feed them. Their incessant nagging could make you even feel depressed or make the healthy food taste like cardboard. You'll start to have doubts that you can succeed with the diet. Just smile and shrug this off. When those feelings happen, then you know that you're winning the battle and the toxic bacteria are dying off. Soon, their abusive manipulation will come to an end and you can control what you eat and how you eat it.

You just must stay strong, especially for the first week. You need to eliminate them and it might be difficult and seem impossible, but you simply cannot give up. Whenever you feel like that craving is going to win, focus on the prize at the end. Get angry if you must! It's not you, not your real body that wants to eat those empty, harmful calories. It's an invasive species of bacteria, one that wants to control you and manipulate you. They want to hurt you and rob you of your precious health. Keep the almonds handy for snacking and if you can't fill the need for sugar, reach for fruit, especially blueberries. You can do it! I promise. You're more than strong enough to survive the cravings.

As you're conquering the bad bacteria, it's time to invite the good bacteria to take up residence. You can do this simply by eating the types of healthy foods that you, and they, can enjoy. You can aid this process as well by drinking probiotic drinks containing Lactobacillus casei. If your gut is a garden, replanting it should start immediately. These drinks are easily found at most health food stores and are becoming easier to obtain. These can also enhance your mood during that difficult first week while you adjust to a healthier diet. And, those salads and beans that were previously bland and flavorless will start to grow in appeal. They'll taste better and you'll find whole grains far more appetizing.

Fast food and sugar will begin to diminish in importance and you will be able to break your dependence. As those bad cravings fade away, it will be easier to eat healthy food because now you'll want to. Healthy foods will taste fantastic. As a bonus, if you do eat sugar after you've transitioned into a healthy diet, your body will respond negatively. You will no longer want to eat it because of how tired and cranky it will make you feel.

CHAPTER 9
The Research Demonstrating the Benefits of an Anti-Inflammatory Vitality Diet

Anyone who has tried to live a healthier lifestyle knows how difficult it can be. Processed, unhealthy foods abound and are often cheaper and seem more accessible than healthy, good-for-you food. Yet our bodies want to be healthy. If we feed them the right fuel, they will maintain a healthy weight and age gracefully. If we feed them chemicals and toxins, the body suffers and there is a higher likelihood of getting sick. The body has to work harder to get rid of those foods, which inflame and irritate it, causing not just the obvious issues like ulcers and digestive issues, but causing inflammation throughout the body that is the cause of everything from cancer to hypertension to Alzheimer's.

These issues don't just make your life harder to live, they are life-threatening and decrease your quality of life. And the only way modern medicine tells you to manage these diseases is with more toxins, in the form of antibiotics, prescription medications and invasive medical treatments. This is so unfortunate! Many medications are toxic in and of themselves and surgeries and traumatic treatments deplete the body of energy. The first prescription you receive should be to eat healthy anti-inflammatory foods!

Healthy eating habits have been shown to significantly reduce the chance of developing a serious condition. For example, eating an anti-inflammatory diet (which includes removing meat from your diet), has been shown to reduce the incidence of heart disease. Why? Because fatty foods like those that most Americans' diets are made up of irritate the heart and make it work harder to pump blood through the body. People who eat an inflammation-fighting diet, however, eat far less fat and almost no unhealthy fat, so their hearts have a much easier time functioning.

In addition, those who eat a healthy diet have higher levels of essential nutrients, including vitamins and minerals. Most people do not realize that their fatigue, weight gain, inability to lose weight, heart problems, digestive issues, etc. are caused by not having enough vitamin C or vitamin D or iron or another vitamin or mineral deficiency.

Studies conducted around these two disparate diets - the typical American or Western diet, that is high fat and carbohydrates and the anti-inflammatory vegetarian diet that is more typical of those living in the East - have found that the Western diet is likely to cause disease, while the anti-inflammatory diet has the potential to prevent and cure disease. Diseases like diabetes and hypertension, both of which are caused by eating an unhealthy diet (that's not just a claim, that's a medical fact), can be prevented and cured by choosing a healthier lifestyle. The range of conditions and diseases that precipitate from just these two diseases or stem from the same underlying causes as diabetes and hypertension are astounding.

For example, most people eat a diet that is high in carbohydrates. While not all carbohydrates are bad, the simple carbs that are easily digested by the body are very bad. They are processed into sugar, which the body easily stores in the form of body fat. The more simple carbs and refined sugars a person eats, the more fat their body will store, even if they are eating relatively few calories. The increase in body fat puts pressure on the heart, joints, lungs, bones, and nervous system. The heart has to pump more blood at a higher pressure. Hypertension (caused by the intake of too much salt and fat), hardens the walls of the veins and arteries, making it more difficult for the body to get blood where it needs to go.

Genetic factors, of course, play a part in all of this, but they are not nearly as important as what kind of fuel you put into your body. Many genetic conditions can be easily controlled when on an anti-inflammatory diet. Research has shown that many of the most common diseases that are managed with expensive medicine (like diabetes) can be better managed simply by changing the way that the patient eats, instead of requiring them to take medication for the rest of their life. A Lanou study found, for example, that type II diabetes is easily managed with a plant-based diet and that those who ate a plant-based diet had a much lower risk of developing diabetes than those who did not eat a vegetarian diet.

Similar studies like the one conducted by the Harvard School of Medicine came to the same conclusion—even going so far as to say that there is a strong connection between eating meat and the risk of developing diabetes, when adjusting for the participants' BMIs, exercise routines, and average caloric intake. Benefits included a lower incidence of cardiac issues. A study specifically considering the effect of eating an anti-inflammatory diet on cardiac health concluded that vegetarians had a 25% lower chance of developing heart disease than meat eater.

Carbohydrates, largely from store-bought bread and other refined, processed sources, are one of the most dangerous parts of the modern diet. They are easily processed into glucose, which spikes the body's blood sugar levels and causes unknown and often dangerous insulin responses. Of course, not all carbohydrates can be classified as "bad", however, the most common carbs eaten are bad.

The refined carbs that most people eat create a cycle of ravenous hunger and fat storage that can be difficult to break out of. Cells will choose glucose over the fat and protein (in the form of muscles) that the body stores. This triggers the person to eat more glucose, which in turn is burned quickly, leaving the person hungry again, even if some of the energy from the food is stored as fat in the body. These spikes and valleys in blood sugar levels can seriously contribute to heart disease.

The anti-inflammatory diet removes sources of glucose, not just sugar, but the refined, simple carbs like potatoes and white flour and white rice from the diet and replaces it instead with foods that have a "low glycemic index." This simply means that they do not have much effect on blood sugar levels. What does someone on the anti-inflammatory diet eat? Beans! And other legumes. Vegetables! And lots more. Any high-fiber whole grain. When most people hear "fiber," they think digestion and that's a great connection to make. The reason high-fiber whole grains are great for digestion is because fiber is very difficult for the body to digest. Don't worry, this isn't a bad thing. This means that you feel fuller longer and that your colon is cleaner and the carbs are not processed into glucose, so your body does not store them as fat.

Another staple of this diet is nuts. Not only do nuts have that low glycemic index that make them perfect for managing diabetes and other blood-sugar related illnesses, they are also a great source of vegetarian protein, are packed with antioxidants, and contain many essential minerals and healthy fats. As long as you are not allergic to walnuts or almonds (two of the best options), these can become a great snack or part of a main dish.

Walnuts are especially high in necessary omega-3 fatty acids. These acids are essential for some of the body's most common functions. They strengthen cells, serve as signals between cells, encourage growth, and moderate inflammation. The alpha linolenic acid that walnuts contain has also been shown to reduce LDL (the bad cholesterol).

Aside from diabetes, which is on the rise in this country, hypertension is another inflammation and Western-diet related illness that can be managed with a steady anti-inflammatory diet. Obesity is one of the leading risk factors for hypertension and the condition is strongly connected to heart disorders. All three of these things can be reduced or eliminated completely by the introduction of a vegetarian anti-inflammatory diet. For example, a study conducted by Sabate and Wien found that someone who switched to an anti-inflammatory diet would lose an average of a pound a week, even if they did not increase their physical activity.

They also confirmed that this kind of diet can be used to lower overall BMI and fight obesity, in adults and children. Studies conducted with children who eat a vegetarian diet are, on average, leaner, than those that eat meat. These studies seem to indicate that both children and adults that eat exclusively plant-based diets have a much better chance of losing weight and keeping it off. They also have lower blood pressure.

That same Lanou study about vegetarian anti-inflammatory diets unveiled an additional positive benefit of these diets one that few people expected or believed could be true. Eating fruits, vegetables, and other plant-based foods can reduce the risk of developing certain cancers. Specifically, areas of the world in which healthy, plant-based diets are more common have much lower rates of breast cancer than areas of the world that eat primarily unhealthy diets. This is because plants contain high levels of phytochemicals which not only prevent cancerous cells from forming, but fight against cancer once it has developed in the body. Vegetarian populations report much lower rates of cancers of the lung and prostate (two of the deadliest forms of cancer). Additional studies indicate that those who cut dairy out of their diets are less likely to develop ovarian cancer and prostate cancer.

The low fat and high fiber structure of a vegetarian diet has been shown to reduce the body's inflammatory response. The strain that chronic inflammation has on a person is tied to everything from cancer to stroke to diabetes. Inflammation is dangerous because it is often invisible and cannot be felt by the person experiencing it. It is a risk factor that is difficult to track, difficult to control, and difficult to understand. An anti-inflammatory diet is specifically designed to eliminate foods from the diet that cause inflammation and to introduce foods that fight inflammation, especially those that contain choline, vitamins D and K, zinc, and betamine.

Plant-based foods are far more likely to contain choline and betamine than a meat-based diet. Besides decreasing inflammation in the body, choline has also been known to improve liver function and can be used by the body to synthesize acetylcholine, which is used by the body as a neurotransmitter, which, in turn, helps to keep the brain healthy and functional and prevent or stave off the development of Alzheimer's disease.

Doctors in mainstream medicine are just now starting to understand how certain diets can be used to affect not just Alzheimer's disease, but also just about every inflammation-related illness or condition. The truth is that until recently, most doctors assumed that diseases were caused by uncontrollable risk factors, including genetics, and that medicine specifically formulated to fight that condition (or, more accurately, its symptoms) were the only way to treat that condition. However, recent studies have shown how nutritional supplements like Souvenaid can help to improve brain function in early-stage Alzheimer's patients. This indicates that proper nutrition earlier in life will not only push back the development of Alzheimer's, but may prevent it.

Returning to cancer, you may not realize that your body will occasionally produce a cancerous cell. Usually, the body's own inhibitors will seek out and destroy the cancer before it starts to multiply. It is only when the body is no longer able to do this that cancer takes hold. People who eat animal proteins are feeding their cancer cells, this specific type of protein encourages the growth of cancer not just by increasing inflammation, but by speeding up cell reproduction rates, while simultaneously making the body acidic.

Those who eat vegetarian diets, however, find that their antioxidant levels are much higher, enabling their bodies to easily neutralize the threat of cancer and fight off free radicals and other toxins in the body that aid in the development of cancer. Fiber, especially, is important in this process, as it scrubs the inside of your body clean. Varied vegetarian diets protect the body, if the individual gets enough protein, as well as fiber, antioxidants, minerals, vitamins, and healthy fats.

Recent studies of breast cancer patients found that those who ate a vegetarian diet had a 25% smaller chance of a new case of breast cancer appearing. Those who had more than five servings of vegetables and fruits every day and who walked at least thirty minutes a day were half as likely to die from cancer as those who did not.

This isn't just true of female cancer patients. In fact, in a study about men fighting heart disease, those that chose a vegetarian diet reversed the progression of the disease. The same was true in a similar study about men battling prostate cancer. While the vegetarian group in both studies steadily improved, the men in the control group who did not choose the vegetarian diet declined.

All this data has been collected by the World Health Organization, which determined that what the American population eat causes about a third of cancer, and it classified mean as a carcinogen. High fat, high sugar foods like meat, dairy, and vegetable oils trigger a woman's body to produce more estrogen. More estrogen means a higher incidence of breast cancer, cervical cancer, and ovarian cancer. The converse is also true, women who eat low fat, low sugar foods produce less estrogen and are less susceptible to cancers in reproductive organs. Across the board, researchers found that those who did not eat meat were less likely to develop whichever disease was being studied.

One good example of a large, sweeping study is the recent study of Seventh-Day Adventists. Adventists have a strict dietary code. They do not smoke or drink and are encouraged to exercise. About half of the entire population of this religion follows a vegetarian lifestyle, while the other half eats some meat. Looking at this group specifically makes it easy to isolate meat eating as a factor, because all other factors are largely the same. A Harvard Medical School study of this group showed that Adventists who did eat meat were about three times more likely to develop colon cancer.

Other studies have backed up this conclusion, showing that processed meat and animal fat, especially that has been cooked, is related to increased cancer risk. For example, studies by the University of Utah, Harvard, the Ontario Cancer Institute, pinpointed cooked red meat, eaten even just once a day, can increase the likelihood of developing cancer by a factor of three. Chicken and pork, are not spared from this same classification, increasing a person's chance of colon cancer also by a factor of three.

An additional study published in the American Dietetic Association Journal found that those who ate red meat more than four times a week were also four times more likely to develop kidney cancer than those who abstained from meat or ate it less than once a week. The study continued to find that those who ate red meat and high-glycemic foods like white bread, rice, and potatoes had a higher risk of cancer even than those who just ate red meat. Pancreatic cancer, one of the deadliest cancers despite being relatively rare, is also more common in meat eaters.

In these studies, cancer is connected to meat eating. Those who did not eat it, had a lower chance of developing cancer. Those who did eat it, a higher chance. The sheer number of studies that have similar results is staggering. Even protracted studies that looked both at vegetarians and meat eaters over the course of their entire lives (conducted by the British Journal of Cancer), say that plant-based diets decreased the likelihood of developing cancer (leukemia, myeloma, lymphoma, breast cancer, etc.) by twelve percent.

But why is this? Red meat stokes cancer's flame, the glutamine present in animal protein acts as food for the cancer cells, along with glucose. Those two together, glucose and glutamate feed cancer cells and allow them to multiply before the body can seek them out. Those who eat diets that are low in glucose and glutamate-producing foods can starve the cancer cells out, preventing them from multiplying.

Studies that have linked glucose to cancer are varied, but one published by the Journal of Clinical Investigation shows how eating glucose can cause cancer. This study was conducted by the China-Cornell-Oxford Project, to determine what caused cancer and similar chronic diseases, how high their mortality rates were, and if diet had any effect on cancer development or mortality rates. They discovered that when Western diets were introduced into areas that ate traditionally Eastern diets, the rates of Western diseases also increased.

What is it about an anti-inflammatory diet that makes it so effective? We've all been told, since we were children, that fruits and vegetables are important. That knowledge is replaced by advertising that shows us how delicious just about everything but fruits and vegetables are. The only food commercial that even mentions a vegetable is for processed salad dressings, which are almost always packed with sugar and unhealthy fats.

The anti-inflammatory diet, however, teaches real nutrition, to ensure the body gets enough zinc, iron, and calcium, vitamins A through E, niacin, fiber, and folates. We may not realize just how damaging not get enough of these nutrients can be. Iron, for example, is essential for ensuring oxygen is properly transported throughout the body. That's why someone who has an iron deficiency is fatigued, because they do not have enough of the mineral their body needs to transport this essential energy-producer throughout the body.

Zinc is another good example. We need zinc to help transport molecules into cells. If you don't have enough zinc, your cells don't get the nutrients they need. We need vitamin A for strong eyes, vitamin E for reproductive health, and vitamin D for strong, resilient bones. When we lack the proper levels of these vitamins, the body gets tired and sick.

Harvard Medical School recommends adding vegetables like bok choy, kale, collards, broccoli, and Chinese cabbage into a diet for proper levels of calcium. But the body doesn't just need calcium. To be able to utilize that calcium, it needs vitamins D and K. It requires potassium and magnesium to transport water, iron to transport oxygen. Eating too much animal protein has been shown to weaken bones, but this can be reversed by increasing calcium and vitamins D and K intake.

THE VITALITY DIET: THE VEGETARIAN/VEGAN ANTI-INFLAMMATORY

The biggest fear most people have as they age is getting sick. Most people equate getting older with getting sicker. That is only true if you have abused your body by not feeding it the right fuel. The inflammation that starts when you are a child and carries through into your adulthood is damaging your system and making you sick. This isn't alternative medicine hokum, this is backed up by scientific research.

Individuals who eat toxin-filled, processed, inflammatory foods do have a higher chance of developing some of the world's nastiest diseases. Even if they don't develop cancer or hypertension or diabetes, they are more susceptible to colds, flus, allergies, and fatigue. On the other hand, those who eat an anti-inflammatory, plant-based diet that is high in phytochemicals and the essential nutrients your body needs, have far lower incidences of those nasty diseases and the everyday illnesses that most people just deal with. Whether you are fighting one of these inflammation-caused diseases (arthritis, cancer, heart disease) or you simply want to prevent them from taking hold later in life, an anti-inflammatory vegetarian diet is the best way to cure or prevent these conditions.

References

Barnard ND, Nicholson A, Howard JL. The medical costs attributable to meat consumption. Prev Med. 1995;24:646-655.

Blaack, EE; Saris, WHM. (1995). "Health Aspects of Various Digestible Carbohydrates". Nutritional Research 15 (10): 1547-73.

Boyd NF, Stone J, Vogt KN, Connelly BS, Martin LJ, Minkin S. Dietary fat and breast cancer risk revisited: a meta-analysis of the published literature. Br J Cancer. 2003;89(9):1672-1685.

Campbell, T. Colin; Chen Junshi; and Parpia, Bandoo. "Diet, lifestyle, and the etiology of coronary artery disease: the Cornell China Study", The American Journal of Cardiology, 82(10), supplement 2, November 1998, pp. 18–21.

Chang-Claude J, Frentzel-Beyme R, Eilber U. Mortality patterns of German vegetarians after 11 years of follow-up. Epidemiology. 1992;3:395-401.

Chang-Claude J, Frentzel-Beyme R. Dietary and lifestyle determinants of mortality among German vegetarians. Int J Epidemiol. 1993;22:228-236.

Chao A, Thun MJ, Connell CJ, et al. Meat consumption and risk of colorectal cancer. JAMA. 2005;293:172-82.

Detopoulou, P., Panagiotakos, D., Chrysohoou, C., Fragopoulou, E., Nomikos, T., Antonopoulou, S., Pitsavos, C. and Stefanadis, C. (2009). Dietary antioxidant capacity and concentration of adiponectin in apparently healthy adults: the ATTICA study. Eur J Clin Nutr, 64(2), pp.161-168.

Dolwick Grieb SM, Theis RP, et al. Food groups and renal cell carcinoma: results from a case-control study. J Am Diet Assoc. 2009;109:656-667.

Giovannucci E, Rimm EB, Stampfer MJ, Colditz GA, Ascherio A, Willett WC. Intake of fat, meat, and fiber in relation to risk of colon cancer in men. Cancer Res. 1994;54(9):2390-2397.

Jenkins, DJ; Jenkins, AL; Wolever, TM; Josse, RG; Wong, GS (1984). "The glycaemic response to carbohydrate foods". The Lancet 324: 388–391.

Lanou, A. (2009). Should dairy be recommended as part of a healthy vegetarian diet? Counterpoint. American Journal of Clinical Nutrition, 89(5), pp.1638S-1642S.

Macdonald, H. (2013). Is ankle strength as important as vitamin D status in helping to prevent falls in winter?. Age and Ageing, 42(2), pp.154-155.

Mehedint, M. and Zeisel, S. (2013). Choline's role in maintaining liver function. Current Opinion in Clinical Nutrition and Metabolic Care, 16(3), pp.339-345.

Murray, A., McMorrow, A., O'Connor, E., Kiely, C., Mac Ananey, O., O'Shea, D., Egaña, M. and Lithander, F. (2013). Dietary quality in a sample of adults with type 2 diabetes mellitus in Ireland; a cross-sectional case control study. Nutr J, 12(1), p.110

Murtaugh MA, Ma KN, Sweeney C, Caan BJ, Slattery ML. Meat Consumption patterns and preparation, genetic variants of metabolic enzymes, and their association with rectal cancer in men and women. J Nutr. 2004;134(4):776-784.

Norat T, Riboli E. Meat consumption and colorectal cancer: a review of epidemiologic evidence. Nutr Rev. 2001;59(2):37-47.

Onodera, Y., Nam, J. and Bissell, M. Increased sugar uptake promotes oncogenesis via EPAC/RAP1 and O-GlcNAc pathways. J Clin Invest. 2014 Jan 2; 124(1): 367–384.

Riccioni, G., Scotti, L., D'Orazio, N., Gallina, S., Speziale, G., Speranza, L. and Bucciarelli, T. (2014). ADMA/SDMA in Elderly Subjects with Asymptomatic Carotid Atherosclerosis: Values and Site-Specific Association. IJMS, 15(4), pp.6391-6398.

Sabate, J. and Wien, M. (2010). Vegetarian diets and childhood obesity prevention. American Journal of Clinical Nutrition, 91(5), pp.1525S-1529S.

Samimi, M., Jamilian, M., Asemi, Z. and Esmaillzadeh, A. (2014). Effects of omega-3 fatty acid supplementation on insulin metabolism and lipid profiles in gestational diabetes: Randomized, double-blind, placebo-controlled trial. Clinical Nutrition.

Scheltens, P., Stam, C., Shah, R., Bennett, D., Wieggers, R., Hartmann, T., Soininen, H., Rikkert, M., Kamphuis, P. and Sijben, J. (2013). The medical food Souvenaid improves memory performance and preserves functional connectivity in mild Alzheimer'/INS;s disease (AD). Journal of the Neurological Sciences, 333, p.e328.

Thorogood M, Mann J, Appleby P, McPherson K. Risk of death from cancer and ischaemic heart disease in meat and non-meat eaters. Br Med J. 1994;308:1667-1670.

Tuso, P. (2013). Nutritional Update for Physicians: Plant-Based Diets. permj, 17(2), pp.61-66.

Willett WC, Stampfer MJ, Colditz GA, Rosner BA, Speizer FE. Relation of meat, fat, and fiber intake to the risk of colon cancer in a prospective study among women. N Engl J Med. 1990;323:1664-1672.

Wolever, Thomas M. S. (2006), The Glycaemic Index: A Physiological Classification of Dietary Carbohydrate, CABI, pg. 65, ISBN 9781845930516. "Sucrose has a low GI because only half of the molecule is glucose and the other half is fructose. So sugars with a low GI are considered to have a low GI primarily because they contain less glucose than starch rather than because they are slowly absorbed."

World Cancer Research Fund. Food, nutrition, physical activity, and the prevention of cancer: A global perspective. American Institute of Cancer Research. Washington, DC:2007.

Part 2: Taking Action

CHAPTER 10
Foods that Heal, Foods that Hurt and Why

Do You Read Food Labels? Here's Why You Should Start.

Two mothers in California recently spearheaded and won a class-action lawsuit against the brand Nutella, because the mothers believed the product was engaged in false advertising. Nutella advertised itself as a "healthy choice" in television commercials, showing mothers giving their children Nutella on wheat toast as a great alternative to sugary breakfast cereals. Of course, Nutella has just as much sugar and far more calories per serving than some of those sugary cereals.

What has made this court case polarizing is the fact that all of Nutella's nutritional facts, including a full list of ingredients, are plainly printed on the product's packaging. Anyone could easily read the information and discover exactly how bad the hazelnut and chocolate spread is. The fact is that too few people read nutritional facts and ingredient lists (and that's why these mothers won the case). If you want to know what's in your food, especially if you are trying to reduce inflammatory foods in your diet, you can't trust advertising, you must read the label, even of products you have been buying for years.

Truly Natural Food Is Not Difficult to Find

Brands know that you want to eat more natural foods. They know that there is a growing movement of individuals and families that want fewer chemicals and more organic products. Because the terms "natural" and "organic" are not heavily regulated, just about any brand can tout themselves as "all-natural" or "organic," when they are still heavily processed and not any better than the "normal" stuff.

Before putting anything that claims to be organic or natural into your shopping cart, turn the box over and read the list of ingredients. Anything that includes high fructose corn syrup, colorants, butylated hydroxytoluene, aspartame, sucralose, saccharin, nitrates, or acesulfame, should go immediately back on the shelf.

Lots of health foods will swap out natural sugar for aspartame or saccharin because they have fewer (or no) calories. They have also, however, been directly linked to cancer and heart disease. There should be a greater distinction between "health" food and "natural foods." Just because something is low in calories doesn't mean it is going to be good for your body.

What to Pick

As you are shopping, look for foods that contain whole, natural ingredients. Brown rice, whole grains, and truly organic vegetables. Living a vegan or vegetarian lifestyle can greatly cut down on the number of additives and chemicals in your diet, as meat is one of the worst offenders, and the replacements are usually some of the best choices you can make including: fresh fruits and vegetables, beans, soybeans, nuts, oats, etc.

What to Avoid

There are specific chemicals that you want to avoid. Besides the ones listed above, be wary of partially hydrogenated oils (trans fats), monosodium glutamate (MSG), fructose, sucrose, and dextrose. Any word that ends in the suffix "-ose" usually refers to an artificial or heavily processed sweetener, that most companies use because they are inexpensive, yet, wreak havoc on the body.

Remember that chemicals can be lurking in anything that has been pre-prepared and packaged. Prepared foods are some of the worst offenders when it comes to chemicals and unnatural additives. Frozen foods, some canned foods, anything that you pull out of a box and bake and microwave is probably going to be laced with preservatives. It is important to note that just because something is "preserved," doesn't necessarily make it bad. Salt is a natural preservative, but most companies use artificial chemicals, rather than salt to preserve foods.

The Bottom Line

If you are trying to reduce your intake of inflammatory foods, it's up to you to filter out the foods that contain chemicals and are being falsely advertised as healthy. You must turn over every box, every can, and read the ingredients list and the nutritional facts. Get to know what kinds of words to look for. In general, anything that you do not recognize or cannot readily pronounce will mean that the product had some sort of artificial ingredient in it.

Take this process seriously if you want to get rid of all inflammatory foods. Don't just trust what it says on the front of the box—verify by reading the entire label. Even things that sound okay, like potassium bromate, can leave deposits of bromide in your system, which can cause cancer (and has caused cancer in lab rats). Don't be duped by the advertising or by the nice natural or organic labels on the box—read the ingredients list and know for certain that what you're eating is free of chemicals, colorants, artificial sugars, and additives.

As I've already covered, there are multiple foods that can help heal your body and restore your health. There are also multiple foods that are, basically, silent killers and saboteurs of your diet.

Food to avoid:

- **Sugars and Artificial Sweeteners** – These do nothing but sabotage you from the moment they cross your lips. If they aren't helping to pack on the pounds by messing with your metabolism, they're changing the way you feel and react to other foods. Think of them as your primary enemy.
- **Processed Foods with Artificial Additives** – They are filled with chemicals, many of which are just as bad, or worse, that sugar. Toss out foods containing MSG, autolyzed yeast, hydrolyzed vegetable protein, BHA, BHT, food coloring like FD&C Red No. 5, glutamate, glutamic acid, parabens, sodium caseinate, mineral oil, etc. Every day they are finding more links between deadly diseases such as cancer and the chemicals that we are ingesting via processed foods.
- **Anything Containing Hydrogenated Oils** – These masked trans fats are considered unhealthy for consumption, yet they are allowed into the food supply by the FDA. Do yourself a favor and avoid them.
- **Masked foods masquerading as something they aren't** – Often you will pick up a food product and realize that you aren't getting what you think you're buying. If you pick up a bottle of green tea, cane sugar shouldn't be in the ingredient list.

- **Coffee** – The caffeine in coffee stresses the adrenal glands, leaving you feeling anxious and causing insomnia. Stress is damaging to the immune system.
- **Dairy** – You should get rid of butter, cheese, ice cream, milk, cream and yogurt. Many people eat yogurt daily as a weight loss food, but yogurt doesn't help you lose weight. You can use sugar-free probiotic yogurt drinks sparingly. Also, cook with olive oil or unprocessed coconut oil - not butter.
- **Yeast** – Do not eat baker's yeast, brewer's yeast, or nutritional yeast. Many people suffer from a candida infection and eating more yeast will aggravate this infection and inflammation. Also, beer, spirits, and wine contain yeast and are difficult for the liver to clean out of your system.
- **Corn** – While corn does contain certain B vitamins and vitamin C, as well as magnesium and potassium, corn is a potential allergen and really doesn't have much nutritional value. Avoid cereal, corn bread, corn chips, and other snack foods made from corn.
- **Peanuts and Rancid Nuts or Seeds** – Peanuts grow underground and may contain mold. They can be potential allergens and rancid nuts and seed contain damaged oils that promote inflammation.
- **Nightshade Vegetables** – Goji berries, eggplants, peppers, paprika, cayenne, jalapeno, potatoes, okra, tomatillos, and tomatoes should not be eaten. The Latin name for this family of plants is Solanaceae, because all of them produce an alkaloid compound called solanine. Solanine is part of these plants' natural defense system, acting as a nerve poison on insects that try to eat the plants. Alkaloids are high in the leaves of nightshades and in the unripe fruit of nightshades like green peppers, green tomatoes and in old potatoes. Tobacco is also a nightshade plant.
- **Meat** - Animal fats have been linked to inflammation in several studies. One tracked how our beneficial gut bacteria change after eating saturated fats and found that as the balance of species shift, it can trigger an immune response that results in inflammation and tissue damage. Saturated fats also contain a compound the body uses to create inflammation naturally called arachidonic acid. Diets lower in this molecule have anti-inflammatory effects and have been shown to improve symptoms in rheumatoid arthritis patients.

Foods to Seek Out

Some foods you want to eat often. These foods can help your body recover and get your hormones in balance, healing you in the process.

- **Fresh Vegetables** – These are a marvelous source of vitamins and minerals. They also help stave off those cravings for sugars and the like by making you feel full and satisfied.
- **Fresh Nuts, Especially Almonds and Walnuts** – These two nuts are loaded in health benefits. Walnuts, in particular, are a source for omega-3 which is essential for hormone balance and to help reduce inflammation.
- **Whole Grains and Legumes** – These are hearty and provide invaluable vitamins and minerals needed to maintain digestion and health overall.
- **Natural Sweeteners** – Agave nectar, brown rice syrup, coconut syrup, raw honey, stevia and yacon syrup are better sweeteners to help you transition to a sugar-free diet.
- **Healthy Oils** – It is best to use avocado, unprocessed coconut, or extra-virgin olive oil and cook using the lowest heat setting possible.
- **Dairy Alternatives** – Use unsweetened almond milk, hemp milk, brown rice milk and small amounts of coconut milk as an alternative to cow's milk.

CHAPTER 11

Beginners Guide to the Anti-Inflammatory Diet: The Basics

If you suffer from an inflammation-related condition or illness, chances are that you've been advised to go on an anti-inflammatory diet. Unlike a diet that is designed to help you lose weight (though that might be a side effect, if you have weight to lose), this diet helps you eliminate the foods that cause inflammation and incorporate the ones that fight it. Here's the basics to getting this diet right:

1. **Go for a fresh variety of foods.** On any diet, it might be tempting to find one food that fits the bill and make it the staple of your meals. Doing that, you're going to get bored, fast. Instead, opt for a wide variety of foods. Keep trying new things.
2. **Eat when you're hungry.** When you're eating a lot of junk food or sugar, you're going to be constantly hungry because you're starving your body. When you're eating a healthy diet, you can eat until you feel full and not gain weight. It's still important to make sure you're getting enough fuel for your body.
3. **Carbs.** It may be surprising to some to learn that you don't have to cut carbs out of your diet entirely - just bread. Women need around 160-200 grams, while men need 240-300 grams. Stick to whole grains, beans, squash, brown rice, and sweet potatoes. Anything that contains high fructose corn syrup is a no-go.
4. **Fat is good.** You need fat to stay healthy. For every one gram of saturated and polyunsaturated fat, you want two grams of monounsaturated fat. Reduce butter, fake cheese with a high fat content, and palm kernel oil. Get more

omega-3 fatty acids from avocados, olive oil, hemp seeds, flax seeds, or a supplement.
5. **Protein.** Most people need in between eighty and one-hundred-twenty grams of protein per day. Get it from beans, and whole-soy foods.
6. **Fiber.** Get forty grams every day. Again, beans are a great option.
7. **Vitamins and minerals.** If you're upping your intake of fruits and vegetables, chances are you're going to be getting the nutrients you need. If not, take an all-natural vegetarian supplement to make sure you're getting the appropriate levels.

This diet doesn't have to be difficult. Follow these guidelines and it's easy!

CHAPTER 12
Great Salads are a Start

It is important to develop daily positive food routines because most of our life is comprised of habit. This is especially true when it comes to eating. People tend to eat breakfast, lunch, and dinner at roughly the same time. They have favorite foods that they crave and keep stocking in their refrigerators. The key to success with the anti-inflammatory diet is creating new habits.

For example, if you aren't in the habit of eating salad for dinner now is the time to start. Great aged balsamic vinegar and deep green unfiltered extra virgin olive oil are essential. Eating for health and weight loss means that you'll be eating a lot of salad greens. I personally usually eat a salad for lunch and dinner. I know what some of you are thinking, salads are boring and that are only so many ways that you can enjoy salad greens. The easiest way to enjoy salads is by using high quality olive oil and aged balsamic vinegar. This combination is my go-to dressing, one that elevates bland greens into something delicious and so good for you. Sure, you might think that you prefer ranch, and you might actually - right now, but it's tremendously unhealthy. You don't want to use it, and most importantly, you don't need it. Also, don't buy just any olive oil or vinegar. These two items will become a central part of your routine, an invaluable asset.

First and foremost, remember one thing when selecting olive oil. Olives are a fruit so settling for less than fresh isn't going to work. Olive oil is a form of fruit juice, at least in a way, and settling for substandard product will yield unhealthful results. It's best to find a farmer, or company, that you can truly trust. Here in California, I can purchase outstanding olive oil right at my local farmer's market. This allows me to not only speak to the farmer directly, but I can also taste the oil prior to purchase. If this isn't an option, especially if you live in a cold weather climate, you may still be able to locate a store that could offer a tasting of select oils. However, be prepared to find a specialty shop or specialized market.

Why a specialty shop? Never ever buy a low-cost bottle of olive oil at a big box grocery store because, again, quality matters. Big box retailers care little about quality and focus on the quantity and profit. I would also recommend staying away from Italian olive oil. You don't know what you're getting if you go the imported route. There are many duplicitous growers in the world. Some growers have even been known to sell what's called "deodorized oil". It's made from olives, so they aren't completely lying to you when they say there is olive oil in the bottle. It's acquired by using the rotten olives, the ones that no one would eat if they saw them in person. The oil itself is initially inedible, but then processed and mixed with other oils is such a way that leaves very few chemical traces. Using this process, it's possible to produce a neutral oil, flavorless and colorless, that can then be mixed with a little of the real stuff and sold as extra virgin oil. That sounds unethical, doesn't it? And it is. However, things can get even worse. Some growers admit to mixing in other oils like safflower with olive oil to cut costs, which is something to look out for if you have a food allergy. You want a single-source oil, not one that has roots in several Mediterranean countries.

If you can't find a local organic olive oil near you, California Olive Ranch produces an excellent extra virgin olive oil that won't disappoint. California Olive Ranch cold presses their 100% California grown olives within hours of picking for a fresher taste and better quality product. Bariani California Olive Oil is also delicious and has the added benefit of being registered as organic. Produced in a limited quantity, Barinai Olive Oil is stone crushed, cold pressed, decanted and unfiltered. That sounds expensive, right? It's affordable, the price on par with most of the big box brands and substitutes.

Once you have a high-quality olive oil, balsamic vinegar is next. You will be tempted to skimp on price here because excellent aged balsamic vinegar is expensive. Resist that temptation and don't be cheap! The plan is to make your salads tasty and healthy so that you'll want to eat them, right? Instead of focusing on the price, try to remember that aged balsamic vinegar is very thick with the consistency of a syrup. You won't need a lot to bring out that "pop" you want from your greens so you can easily expect a $40 bottle to last between two and four months. That averages out to roughly a few quarters a salad. The secret when purchasing balsamic vinegar is that you want to get it aged. Why? Because the longer it ages, the tastier, sweeter it becomes. If you can't find a reasonable version locally, Villa Manodori Balsamic Vinegar is a wonderful alternative. It is made in limited quantities from trebbiano grapes grown in Modena

Italy. Also, it is aged for a minimum of 10 to 15 years and it is simply fantastic. Another thing you must do is avoid anything with the phrase "balsamic glaze". It may appear thick and sweet like aged balsamic vinegar, but that is achieved cheaply with additives you don't want to eat. Instead, perfectly aged balsamic vinegar as well as an outstanding extra virgin olive oil will give you the ability to create a delicious salad, one that you want to eat.

CHAPTER 13
Stay Hydrated and Restore Alkalinity to Your Body

Another indispensable way to regain your health is to restore the alkalinity to your body. To do this I drink a large glass of filtered water mixed with fresh organic lemon juice. I always do this first thing when I get out of bed. Another great drink is made by adding a shot of apple cider vinegar. You can take apple cider vinegar as a shot, but the taste is quite strong, so it would be wise to mix it with water or with the lemon juice/water mixture.

You're probably thinking, 'how can adding acid restore alkalinity?' It's all part of the way our bodies work. Unfortunately, the typical western diet creates an almost overwhelmingly acidic bodily pH and the resulting problems are numerous. Apple cider vinegar has an amazing impact on our pH levels. That effect (increased alkalinity) plays a large part in its healing properties. Studies have shown that apple cider vinegar can potentially cure, or help manage, allergies, acne, cholesterol, weight loss, arthritis, fatigue, and the list goes on. It can also be used to improve insulin sensitivity for people suffering from type 2 diabetes and help dissolve kidney stones. Apple cider vinegar does this by reacting with the toxins in our bodies, turning them into more controllable, much less toxic substances.

One thing to point out with apple cider vinegar is that you don't want the general, cheap apple cider vinegar. All the health benefits are linked exclusively to the "mother" that is present in raw, organic apple cider vinegar. Most filtered brands have removed this essential part, rendering it almost useless. The "mother" is where the nutrients, raw enzymes, and the GI friendly bacteria live. Filtered, clear brands, lack this part. The price is somewhat higher; however, it is not astronomical and my preferred brand, Bragg's, is especially reasonable and often found in most grocery stores. Spend the extra money because you're worth it.

You've heard this a thousand times, but I'm going to tell you again that you should be drinking lots of clean, fresh water. Maintaining proper hydration will help remove toxins from your body. As a rule of thumb, divide your body weight in half and drink that many ounces of healthful liquid per day. That means men should consume about 128 ounces of water daily, and women should consume about 88 ounces. Other beverages like herbal teas, as well as the moisture content of foods, also count toward your water intake. If you get even a hint of thirst, grab a glass of water. You need it.

I know that you're thinking that you might want to drink something else other than water, lemon water, or vinegar water. Of course, you do! There are several options. I occasionally indulge in small amounts of organic soy milk (non-GMO), rice milk, coconut milk, or even oat milk. You should be careful with these types of drinks, because many manufacturers add sugars and flavors, increasing the risk of inflammation. Another thing to look out for is an ingredient called "carrageenan". Many makers of organic foods add this, citing that it is indeed organic and vegan. However, it has been linked to cancer promotion and other ill effects, some of which make it easy to place in the "avoid at all costs" column. Not to mention, it's been linked to inflammation which is what you are trying to avoid. If you are a coffee drinker, and many of us are, Teeccino Herbal coffee can satisfy that craving. It's caffeine free and helps to restore alkaline balance.

CHAPTER 14

10 Easy Ways to Drink More Water for Weight Loss

There's a reason you can go a month without food but only three days without water—it's essential for every single process in the body. Besides just keeping us alive, water can help you lose weight, get clearer skin, and even achieve a positive mood. You are encouraged to drink at least eight glasses of water a day. If you're not getting your quota, here are ten ways to get more water into your day:

1. **Flavor your water.** If you find water boring, you can easily make it more alluring by flavoring it. There are plenty of water flavorings you can buy at stores, but go natural and use some lemon, some orange, or some mint in a fruit infusion bottle.
2. **Spice up your food.** The spicier your food, the more water you'll drink. Salt has the same effect, but spicy foods get you to drink more water, without the negative side effects of eating too much salt. Plus, spicy foods kick your metabolism into high gear.
3. **App it.** You can download an app on any platform (iOS, Android, and Windows), that lets you track how much water you've drank and can even remind you to drink more.
4. **Get a water filter.** If your tap water tastes nasty or is full of chemicals, a water filter is a great investment. I use a reverse osmosis system.
5. **Keep it on you.** You're more likely to drink water throughout the day if you carry a water bottle with you.
6. **Take it to the gym.** Just drinking out of the water fountain isn't going to cut it. Bring your own bottle.

7. **Be more economical.** Most restaurants don't charge for a glass (and unlimited refills) of water. Even if they do charge, it's not going to be anywhere near as expensive as soda or alcohol.
8. **Snack on fruits or veggies.** While chomping on celery, melons, or cucumbers might not feel like you are hydrating, they can help hydrate your body.
9. **Think of it like a weight loss supplement.** Drinking a full glass of water before you start to eat can help you feel fuller, faster, which means you'll eat less at dinner.
10. **Alternate water and wine.** You shouldn't drink any alcohol if you want to heal your body. However, if you are going to drink, wine is the best option. Alternating water and wine on your fun night out will keep you from getting too dehydrated (and keep you from getting a hangover), and will prevent you from drinking too much.

CHAPTER 15

Detox Your Home and Throw The Poisons Out!

The home is where most people spend the majority of their life, even if the largest amount of time spent at home is spent sleeping. This means that most the air that we breathe is the air in our homes. Luckily, unlike the air at the office, mall, grocery store, or street, we can control the air in the home. If you are ready to detox your home, here are ten easy ways to do it:

1. **Clean your flooring.** Vacuum regularly. It might not be your favorite chore (though with headphones and some tunes, why can't it be fun?), but it will help eliminate much of the dust in your home. Clean your linoleum, tile, or lacquered wood floors with a mixture of hot water and vinegar, to skip the harsh, volatile chemicals.
2. **Clean your glass.** Windows and mirrors are two other areas where dust can accumulate. That hot water and vinegar mixture will work for glass surfaces, too.
3. **Clean your toilets, tub, or shower.** These are germ hotspots. A half cup of white vinegar and a fourth of a cup of baking soda in a gallon of water will disinfect without the chemicals.
4. **Naturally Polish your furniture.** While unpolished furniture won't add toxins your home, trying to polish them with store-bought products will. Use a little olive oil and lemon juice instead.
5. **Bring some outside in.** Plants of all kinds are natural air filters.
6. **Change filters in air conditioners and furnaces.** Especially right before their first use, but any time your home starts to smell or feel musty, change those filters.

7. **Take off your shoes before entering the house.** This will keep anything you pick up in your errands or at work outside the home.
8. **Choose your candles wisely.** Candles can be a great way to incorporate some aromatherapy into your daily routine, but make sure they aren't petroleum-based (paraffin). Soy or beeswax is much better.
9. **Choose clay paint.** If you can find it, paint your rooms with clay paint, instead of toxic oil or lead paint. It's hypoallergenic and can absorb toxins out of the air.
10. **Read your labels.** Even if something says it's all-natural, do your research before buying anything. Lots of brands market themselves as green and/or natural, when it's just the same toxic cleaner in a different bottle.

The Kitchen

Your kitchen is most likely filled with processed foods. No, they're not just merely processed, but processed to the point that they are no longer food. Your cupboards and cabinets are packed with chemicals instead of vegetables and grains, vegetables in cans that have been exposed to preserving agents like BPA that cause cancer. If you're daring enough to read the list of ingredients on your staple foods, most likely you'll be shocked and a little bit disgusted by what you see. Probably sugar in everything, lots of hydrogenated oils, and unknowables. If you don't know what an ingredient is - DON'T EAT IT. Google it. It may be fine, but it may be toxic. You cannot count on the FDA to protect you against toxic ingredients.

Look, if you have unhealthy food in your kitchen part of you will want to consume it out of sheer habit, not to mention the ease of access. You need to rid yourself of it, removing them from sight and your kitchen. This will make your kitchen healthier and safer and can remove some of the challenges of taking up a new healthy diet. If you stock your pantry with vegetables and healthy snacks like almonds and then replenish your fridge with fresh fruits and healthy drinks, you'll indulge in them. Yes, eat an entire carton of organic blueberries in one sitting!

Stop buying junk. I know that sounds simple, but in the grocery store that bright packaging is going to call to you. It's how marketing firms earn their bread, after all. They want to sell you those chemicals and additives and they want you to crave them. They know exactly what they're doing. Think of that impulse, last minute section at the grocery stores and super markets. Have you ever seen vegetables or fruit cups lined up next to the conveyer belt? No, but you'll see candy and sugar laden soda. Also, like mom said, don't shop when you're hungry. People have a hard time thinking straight when they're hungry, because a more primitive part of our brains becomes active.

Here are some steps to help you along your journey to detoxify your kitchen area.

Step 1: Set aside a time, a day, and an hour to begin the kitchen clean up.

- You need to specify a time to begin because, though it may sound simple in nature, you're going to need to dive deep into food labels to get to the bottom of what's a good food and what's a bad food. If you feel too guilty about throwing away all this "food", then you'll need containers as well because there is always a way to make use of food if you no longer need it. Several charities will accept canned goods. If nothing else, have a bag nearby so that, if you can't "rehome" those foods, you can at least recycle their packaging.

Step 2: You'll need to scrutinize and analyze those labels as completely as you can. This won't apply to fresh foods, of course, but if you do insist on some canned or prepared items, you have to be diligent about reading their ingredient labels.

- Focus on the ingredients and not the nutritional facts chart. You can have a soda with 0 calories and that doesn't make it healthy. There are chemicals and additives in most processed and canned food. If there were no chemicals the food would rot. You have to look for those chemicals because they are toxic. Don't get caught up on calories. Go straight for the ingredients list.
- If you can't pronounce it, toss it. If it sounds like something from high school chemistry class, you really don't want to eat it.
- Pay careful attention to the order of the ingredients as well. They are listed in order of what is most abundant down to what is the smallest amount. Fruit juice with the first ingredient of corn syrup or sugar going to be mostly sugar. The first ingredient, after all, is the weightiest of the ingredients. That's something to consider carefully while examining the labels.
- Throw away products with sugar, corn syrup, corn sweetener, crystalline fructose, dextran, Diastatic malt powder, diastase, Ethyl Maltol, cane juice, galactose, Glucose, Lactose, Maltodextrin, Maltose, Panela, and others.
- If it has a marketing ploy like the Kellogg's Corn Flakes 2-Week Weight Loss Challenge on the front of the box, odds are that you don't need it. It's usually a sure sign that it's there to simply trick you into purchasing their product.

Seeing these labels will make you think "healthy" but in reality they are anything but. Health bars and sports drinks fit into this category. The additives erase any benefits they may have.

Step 3: Now that you know what to look for, it's time to ditch those foods. Simple as that. Donate or recycle what you can and remove it from your sight and your reach.

Sugar is a huge culprit when it comes to creating havoc on your health. Hidden sugars lurk everywhere, from cereals to wheat products and many of these hide under the illusion of being healthy. And it truly is an illusion. Sugar can go by hundreds of different names in ingredient labels, masking it and allowing your eyes to simply not recognize what you're reading. There are 257 names for sugar in food. It's often derived from corn and accompanies things like maltodextrin or xantham gum. It will make you fat and it will make you crave it as surely as any addiction. Condiments are often overlooked means by which sugar gets into your diet. Salad dressings, ketchup, or barbecue sauce are often sugar bombs.

And remember, don't be afraid of fats. Not all fats are bad or hazardous and some are good for you. Fat, in and of itself, doesn't make you fat. However, bad fats can cause your metabolism loads of trouble. One easy way to jumpstart removing the bad fats is to throw away, or give away, any highly refined cooking oils you might have. Corn and soy oils in particular. You should just stick with a high quality organic extra virgin olive oil. Any fried foods you may have in your freezer were most likely prepared with the bad fat so they will need to go as well. Margarine, shortening, both are sources of "bad fat". They are loaded with trans-fat that not only creates inflammation in your body, but has been linked to the development of heart disease. Be on the lookout for this keyword: hydrogenated fat or hydrogenated anything. That's a fancy term for trans-fat, another trick of marketing to make you think it's something innocuous. The U.S. FDA announced in 2013 that partially hydrogenated oils (PHOs), the primary dietary source of artificial trans-fat in processed foods, are not 'generally recognized as safe' for use in food.

And while sugar is a culprit, so are artificial sweeteners. Aspartame, sucralose, Splenda, NutraSweet, these artificial sweeteners are just chemicals. If it ends in "ol", such as sorbitol, just toss it. This extends to sugar alcohols as well. You don't want or need them in your diet. Stevia is slightly better in this regard, but only the whole plant extract-like NuNaturals liquid Stevia. Pure Via and Truvia are examples of Stevia that are merely chemical extracts of the source plant. I call it "faux Stevia". Regardless, use it sparingly. There is research into other sources of healthier sweeteners, but anything sweet is going to make you hungry. Not to mention that sweetness can lower your metabolism and help store body fat. When you look in your fridge, you should see fresh foods in their natural unprocessed state.

If it looks how it grows, then eat it!

CHAPTER 16

Anti-Inflammatory Essentials: What You Should Always Have In Your Kitchen

Once you've removed the offending foods from your cupboard and your fridge, it's time to replace them with healthy, nutritious alternatives. You want fresh foods and you want things that you can grab that will satisfy your cravings.

1. Vegetables are a freebie. The non-starchy kind, of course. You can eat as many as you would like, as often as you would like. Don't go hungry, because your metabolism shuts off if you starve yourself. When you eat salads and fresh vegetables, you shouldn't have a moment's guilt. You'll need to watch your fruit intake, because fruits do contain fruit sugar like fructose and too much fruit sugar will increase your insulin levels. When it comes to fruit, berries should be your star. They contain a wealth of antioxidants that can help build a healthier you. Also, remember that, if possible, to shop for organic locally grown produce. If you look for seasonal food, you will get better deals and purchase more of it as a result. To get a started, visit your local farmer's market this week. I go to the farmer's market every Tuesday and Saturday. There you can make good food choices and even ask the grower questions about how to prepare the produce and recipes.

2. Don't be afraid of dry unprocessed foods. They have a much longer shelf life and can include a variety of items. Roasted or raw nuts, and legumes will fall into this category. Don't forget to try quinoa and gluten-free grains as well. You can find brown rice, quinoa, barley, lentil beans, almonds and more in the bulk food section of the grocery store. You'll need to grab a bag and write down the number of the food item to show the store clerk at checkout.

THE VITALITY DIET: THE VEGETARIAN/VEGAN ANTI-INFLAMMATORY

   Having lots of healthy dry goods at home will be the foundation for most healthy anti-inflammatory recipes.
3. Variety is the spice of life and that is especially true when it comes to stocking your seasonings and spices. They are used sparingly so a small container can last a very long time. If possible, again, shop for organic. Also make sure the labels don't indicate any hidden, nasty ingredients. Look out for sugar and corn syrup, as well as chemical enhancements. Good examples of stable spices include: sea salt, fresh black peppers, turmeric, cumin, ginger, and chili powder.
4. Fresh foods are also a given. You don't want something that has been frozen with additives to "stabilize" it. You want fresh vegetables and, if need be, frozen vegetables. Also, if you purchase canned items, make sure the label says the lining of the can is BPA free.

It may sound limiting at first, but you'll get the hang of healthy eating and soon you'll look back on what you used to eat and ask yourself, "Why did I think all that crap tasted good?!"

CHAPTER 17
Pills and Supplements: What to Look For

If you're trying to live a healthier lifestyle, you are probably also using supplements to make sure that you are getting all the nutrients that you need. While supplements can be a great way to make sure your body has exactly what it needs, not all supplements are created equal. You may be shocked when you turn the bottle over and read what is in those supplements, despite being labeled "organic" or "natural" or "100% safe" on the front of the bottle. The plain truth is that supplements can contain toxins, just like anything else produced and processed by the food industry.

Of course, there are plenty of honest companies that are producing supplements that are 100% safe to use and contain no toxins. To tell the difference between who is being honest and who is lying, you must look for those toxins and that starts with knowing what ingredients are dangerous. Here are just ten of the most common toxins added to supplements:

1. **Aluminum (in high levels)** – Aluminum itself isn't necessarily bad for you. You need small amounts of aluminum to survive, but many supplements will have massive amounts of this metal, which can be extremely dangerous. You may be familiar with a recent scandal in the health foods industry, where one detox liquid was recalled because it had more than 1200ppm of this metal.
2. **Maltodextrin** – This is one of the most common toxins added to supplements, and it is usually extracted right from GM corn. It's a starch that has been genetically modified, which is never good for your body. If you are looking for a supplement, look for one that contains tapioca maltodextrin, which is more likely to be organic and non-genetically modified. Better yet, look for a product that contains no maltodextrin at all.

3. **Inorganic minerals** – If you are buying cheap vitamins, you are likely just spending money on capsulated scrap metal. You probably heard news stories recently about tests done on vitamin supplements that found that a surprising number of them were filled with sand. Yes, sand. While they might be trying to pass that sand off as calcium (which can be derived from seashells, but not in a form that your body can use), it is just sand. Magnesium, when sold in an oxide formulation, is completely useless to your body. Iron capsules? Probably just iron filings—again, not useful to your body. If you are trying to get the right levels of vitamins and minerals, it's best just to increase your organic plant intake.
4. **Lead and arsenic** – Some of the most unscrupulous companies in the health food industry will source their herbs from China. What's wrong with China? Besides being the country that owns most of our national debt, China is also home to the most pollution in the world. Heavy metals—the scary ones—are surprisingly high in herbs sources from China, including mercury, arsenic, lead, and cadmium. And they don't perform any kind of testing before exporting the herbs, so there is no way to know if they have been tainted. Look for brands that source their herbs from other Western countries, please.
5. **Acrylamides** – This is a chemical most commonly found in heavily processed and fried foods, but not one you'll find listen in the ingredients. Why? Because it's not actually intentionally added to the food. It is a compound created during the frying process, and they significantly increase your risk of developing cancer. But if you don't eat processed chips or other fried foods, how can these get into your system? They are also found in products like prune juice and breakfast cereal. These may be impossible to completely avoid, even in the best supplements, but you should know that vitamin C can combat this chemical effectively.
6. **Vitamin C (derived from GM corn)** – If you see something that says it contains ascorbic acid that probably means that any vitamin C that it contains is from GM corn.

Most manufacturers test their own products and provide the reports to their retailers and vendors, but not to the public. Essentially, they can lie all they want about what their products contain, and you might never know. Look for a supplement from a company that has engaged with independent testing—this is a good sign they're being honest about what their products contain.

CHAPTER 18

What Is The Difference Between Omega-3 And Omega-6?

It is vitally important to control inflammation through consumption of omega - and omega-6. When a person's intake of omega 6 fats exceeds their intake of omega 3 fats, as is often the case in the typical Western diet, increased inflammation can result. Omega-3 and omega-6 are both types of essential fatty acids. We can't make them by ourselves but they are essential to everyone's bodily function. The only way to obtain them is through introducing certain foods into our diet. They might sound similar due to both having the same type of fat (polyunsaturated), but they differ slightly due to their chemical structure.

Omega-3 is often found in walnuts or flaxseed, and omega-3 eggs. The purpose of seeking out and obtaining this particular fatty acid is that it contains two critical components that the body relies on. The first of these, eicosapentaeonic acid, is also called EPA for short. The second, docosahexaenoic, or DHA, works with EPA to help build hormones. They are also important for the immune system and its continued functionality, as well as helping with the clotting of blood and growth and regrowth of cells.

Omega-6, has multiple readily available sources. It is found in seeds and nuts and, fortunately, still present in the oils extracted from them. That is fortunate because the body constructs hormones from present or available omega-6 fats. These hormones work in conjunction with those obtained from the omega-3 variety, having opposite effects and impacts on the body. Omega-6 is extremely useful and necessary for the act of inflammation. While that sounds bad (especially considering the nature of this book) remember that inflammation is an important part of the immune system. Along with this important function, it aids in cell proliferation as well as blood clotting. Omega-3, conversely, decreases those functions and keeps things balanced and functional. Without the two working together, things become lopsided and inefficient. The produced hormones simply must be in balance in order to maintain your health.

Due to the limited sources of omega-3 fats, often our hormones are out of balance. Scientists have long hypothesized that these limited resources and the imbalance it brings are the contributing factor to many diseases such as asthma and cancer. In that same classification, many autoimmune diseases and rampant inflammation could be controlled with healthy intakes of omega-3. This imbalance is also potentially to blame for the rise in obesity and depression and any of the other emotional fallouts of having a hormonal imbalance. One study even attributed violence to this imbalance. In that study, Dr. Joseph Hibbein found that violence dropped in a British prison by an astounding 37 percent when omega-3 oils were added to the diets of prisoners.

Omega-6 fats do have a place in a healthy diet, yet given their widespread occurrence in the food supply very little attention needs to be made in obtaining these essential fatty acids. Instead, it is important to reduce omega-6 fats, while increasing omega-3 fats. This can contribute to a healthier ratio of these fats.

You can reduce your consumption of omega-6 by cook with olive or flax oil, and by taking supplements that contain only omega-3 fats (EPA/DHA).

Most nutritionists recommend taking up to 2000mg of EPA and 2000mg of DHA daily as a general supplement. Some arthritis researchers are recommending up to 2600mg a day with the Arthritis Foundation suggesting that the daily dosage be 3000mg twice a day for maximum benefit.

CHAPTER 19
Research Shows You May Not Be Losing Weight Because You Need Vitamin D

Vitamin D is one of the most important nutrients in our diet and many people do not get enough, especially if you are allergic to milk, stay out of the sun to avoid sunburn and skin cancer, or are a vegan. While our bodies can produce vitamin D, it is only produced when the skin is exposed to sunlight. It's also only naturally available in a very few foods, many of which you might have to avoid because of allergies, intolerances, or other diet restrictions.

This leaves a huge portion of the population vitamin D deficient, which in turn has several very negative side effects, including the development of cancer, serious skeletal system issues like rickets, asthma, cardiovascular diseases, and many more. One of the most common side effects of a vitamin D deficiency is weight gain or an inability to gain weight. Why? Because every single cell, from your brain to the blood vessels in your feet needs vitamin D. If you don't have enough to go around, your body will sense the deficiency and react.

In this case, because vitamin D plays a big role in how much fat your body stores and how much it burns, it will react by storing fat. When you get enough vitamin D, either by upping your intake of D-rich foods or by taking a vitamin D supplement, the vitamin tells the body it's time to start burning excess fat, not storing it. But why does this happen?

It probably dates to our earliest human ancestors. Because vitamin D is so necessary for every process in the body, if you aren't getting enough, the body thinks it is not getting enough nourishment and it goes into survival mode. It starts storing fat to use a fuel in the future, because it thinks a famine is ahead.

But the causes go even deeper than that. Vitamin D can help turn off cravings and hunger. It can boost your brain's production of serotonin (the feel-good chemical), and it even makes sure that other vitamins and minerals are being properly processed by your body—especially calcium. It might be time to consider taking a vitamin D supplement to make sure you switch off your body's famine response and start losing weight!

An Australian study found that taking 500 mg of nicotinamide (a form of vitamin D3) twice a day cut the occurrence of basal cell and squamous cell carcinomas by 23 percent among 386 Australians who already had had at least two of these skin cancers during the previous five years. The average number of earlier skin cancers among study participants was eight, although one patient reported 52 cases. Study participants who were randomly assigned to take daily B3 averaged 1.77 new cancers during the year-long study, compared with 2.42 cases among participants who received a placebo. The patients who took D3 also had fewer cases of actinic keratosis, skin thickenings that can become malignant. Lead researcher Diona Damian said the protective effects of D3 didn't continue after people stopped taking it.

CHAPTER 20
The Gym Isn't As Important As You Think It Is

I used to believe that going to the gym was the only sure way of combating weight gain. I tried for the longest time to work out every day. Sadly, I kept eating inflammatory foods and going to the gym did little to help me on my journey to weight loss and health.

The truth is, no matter how much you are in the gym, or how long you work out, if your body is inflamed and at war with itself, you won't begin to make a dent in your weight and you will continue to suffer from poor health. Building muscle and helping to strengthen your heart and lungs is of course beneficial. However, if you neglect your diet, and especially your GI tract, you're fighting a losing battle.

It's true that muscle helps burn fat and strength is, basically, power, but even if you build muscle, fat is going to continue to be stored and stockpiled by your unhealthy immune/digestive system.

Of course, you should continue to walk or exercise regularly. Getting off the couch is important, but it isn't the main thing. Combined with a healthy diet, regular exercise will escalate and advance your transition into better health, but it can't do it alone. You must remember that. You'll still have to make dietary changes to get ahead and achieve that goal that you desperately want.

CHAPTER 21

Stop Counting Calories! Why Calorie Counting Won't Help You Lose Weight

When most people first try to lose weight, they usually start by counting their calories. Whether they immediately reduce their caloric intake, just start paying attention to how many calories they are eating (which can sometimes be a shocking number), or actively plan every single calorie they eat, most people do not realize that this simply will not help.

Why? Well, there are many reasons. To start, the calorie counts listed on every package of food sold aren't even *correct*. Sure, it lists how many calories that food contains, but it doesn't tell you how many calories you get out of the food. That means if you are trying to lose weight by reducing your caloric intake, you still will have no idea how many calories you are eating. We're told a calorie is an equal unit of energy no matter what type of food it comes from, but if you're eating toxic food; your body will react in an entirely different way than if you are eating healthy food.

Processed Food and Calories

When food is processed, which you can do in your home or can occur in some food factory, it is far more difficult to determine how those calories will affect you. Processed food is cooked, blended, refined, and often laced with chemicals, additives and fillers. All that cooking and lacing changes how many calories your body gets from the food and what it does with those calories.

For example, if you eat raw carrots, you will lose more weight than if you eat cooked carrots. Why? Because cooking and all types of processing changes how food affects your body. Cooking is a type of processing. In the food industry, most of the food that makes it to the shelves has been far more processed than simply being cooked.

When you think about this from an evolutionary standpoint, it makes a little bit more sense. When our ancient ancestors finally discovered fire, and learned to cook their food, they gained more energy from it, meaning that their bodies digested more of the food and therefore utilized more of the calories. Those extra calories are partially to thank for our big brains and relatively large bodies (our evolutionary ancestors were much smaller). Cooking food is part of what made us humans bigger with smarter brains, the strength to bear more children, and the ability to travel with pre-cooked food that would not spoil-all aided in our evolutionary development.

The more processed something is (despite what kind of calories it contains; carbs, protein, fats) the easier it is for your body to digest and synthesize energy from it, but this is not always a good thing. If you are sitting at a computer for most of the day and not burning off all that energy, your body will simply store it. That means that the more processed a food is, the more weight you will gain.

When food has just been cooked, and is warm, it is usually easier to digest. With some types of food, like those containing starch, if it has been cooked and then cooled, the starch solidifies to the point that it resists digestion and will be passed out of your body, rather than burned for energy. That makes cold beans, eaten the next morning for a hurried breakfast, better in terms of weight lose than hot beans eaten the night before. I'm not telling you to only eat uncooked raw food, although some people do. I'm sharing this information with you so that you can make a more informed decision about what to eat when you're trying to lose weight.

Softer Food Makes You Gain Weight

The easier a food is to chew, the more calories your body will be able to extract from it. If you're running a marathon tomorrow, that makes a protein smoothie a good option, as your body will be able to easily get the energy it needs. However, in our everyday lives, this usually means that our bodies are first, getting more energy than they need, and second, not working very hard to get that energy. It is much more difficult to digest a raw carrot than it is to digest a cooked one, because the cooking has already done half of the body's work. You will still lose weight with healthy anti-inflammatory smoothies, but you may lose it in a more gradual manner.

In 2013 researchers at Department of Nutrition Sciences, Graduate School of Health and Nutrition Science, Nakamura Gakuen University, Japan conducted research on lab rats and found that even when fed the same weight and number of calories, rats who ate soft, puffy food gained more weight, faster, than rats that ate solid, denser food. They concluded that the rats eating softer food did not have to work very hard to digest that food, so they utilized more of the calories, and those that ate harder food, had to work harder, and therefore utilized fewer calories.

The Bottom Line
You can't trust the food label; even extremely accurate calorie counts will not tell you how much energy you are actually getting from the food and whether or not it will be stored by your body as fat or actually used. If you are looking to lose weight, you shouldn't be counting calories, you should be focusing on eating an anti-inflammatory diet.

Part 3: The World and You

CHAPTER 22
If Slow is Good for Food, Why Not Medicine?

The slow food movement, besides cutting out a big portion of the junk food that is seriously bad for us, encourages its followers to think carefully and deeply about the food that they eat. It's not just about getting full as quickly as possible, but filling your body with delicious, nutrient-rich food, instead of wreaking havoc like most junk food does. Why can't the concept be the same for medicine?

Medicine and our opinion about medicine has largely gone the same way as our cultural opinion about food. It should work quickly and well; despite whatever side effects it might have. It's all about technology and the "industry" of medicine, and less about what makes the patient better, and not just better in the short term, but healthier overall. It sounds like a conspiracy theory to say that Big Pharma wants us to be sick, but if we weren't reliant on Z-Packs and cough syrup and chemotherapy, how would they make their money?

We want our healthcare to be fast, because being sick or hurt is uncomfortable and it interrupts our daily lives, making it difficult or sometimes impossible to work, spend time with family, or pursue the hobbies and activities that make life worth living.

But fast medicine often means inaccurate or haphazard treatments. For example, have you ever been to the emergency room for something urgent, but not necessarily life threatening? Depending on which ER you go to and which doctor you get, you might find yourself have an abdominal CT scan when you came in for a sinus infection. That's not always the case, but many doctors, especially those in busy wards or offices, will often order all tests that seem relevant, even if both the patient and the doctor have a pretty good idea of what the problem is.

Slow medicine, on the other hand, means that both doctors and patients (and all other healthcare professionals) have a more active hand in healthcare. Exams and observation should be more deliberate. Patients, especially, must be willing to speak up, tell their doctor the truth, and recognize that most of the medicines on the market today do not (and are not designed to) work perfectly and completely—they are designed to work quickly. Slow medicine means giving up the idea that there is some sort of "magic bullet" that can solve a health problem, and understanding that lasting lifestyle changes are often a much better solution than a pill or a shot.

CHAPTER 23
Policies to Make the World a Healthful Planet

Healthy nutrition is essential, beginning with fetal development and continuing through infancy, childhood, adolescence, and all stages of adulthood into the elder years. When it comes to considering the later years in life, you must consider the long-term impact that nutrition can have. We know about the origin of disease and the connection to aging, and therefore it is appropriate to become focused on the beginning stages of life to get a jumpstart in health for our golden years.

We need healthy communities and healthy workplaces to truly thrive. Some communities are "food deserts" without access to fresh foods and where the idea of a farmer's market is alien. This needs to change. All government programs should prioritize nutrition early on, earmarking healthy items and focusing on educating the public at large rather than just ignoring the problem. Food stamps, often the only source of food for many low-income workers, should offer up a way to obtain healthier, more nutritious items rather than the bargain boxes of macaroni and chemical cheese.

Emphasizing the importance of breastfeeding should also be a priority, combined with concerted efforts to improve overall infant nutrition. Making baby, or toddler, food at home can eliminate the toxic additives that can lead to an unhealthy body at the very beginning of life. Employers should support and encourage breastfeeding after the mothers return to work.

Nursing homes and schools often offer bad nutritional choices. Sadly, many of the affected people don't have the ability to speak for themselves. These foods are bought in bulk based on price with no real attention paid to ingredients. Our reliance on fossil fuels is disheartening and the chemicals we spray our foods with is more than a little disturbing. Fortunately, the world is waking up and realizing that we are not only poisoning our planet, but we're also poisoning ourselves.

CHAPTER 24

Research Shows How Chiropractic Care Helps Weight Loss

One of the most common misconceptions about chiropractic care is that it's only for athletes and people with serious skeletal problems. The truth is that chiropractors can help with a range of problems and that their treatments can align more than just your joints and spine. Many people who have been overweight visit chiropractors to help realign the body after years of carrying excess weight. But did you know that regular alignments can help you lose the weight in the first place?

While alignments do not take the place of diet and exercise and nothing can when it comes to sustained, maintainable weight loss incorporating chiropractic care into your weight loss strategy can ensure that you lose more weight, faster. Losing any amount of weight can drastically change your body, and some people find that getting adjusted throughout the process can make it less painful and dangerous to lose weight.

Many chiropractors can also offer nutritional counseling and expert advice about what kinds of workouts are best not just for losing weight, but for building the muscles that you need to stay healthy throughout the weight loss process. Many general practice doctors can offer you some suggestions and some general nutritional guidelines, but chiropractors are usually experts in the scientific balance of the body achieving it and maintaining it.

Another one of the benefits of working with a chiropractor is having another knowledgeable voice and source of encouragement. Most people find weight loss more manageable when they take a varied approach, rather than just cutting calories or just adding in exercise.

Especially at the beginning of the weight loss process, it can be painful to exercise. Sharp pains in the knees or back are common complaints and often an excuse many people use to skip a day or stop working out altogether. Your joints and muscles might not be used to the strain. If the pain persists, as it often does, a chiropractor can help to alleviate it, which means workouts are more enjoyable, or at the very least, not as painful.

And when your body is properly aligned, it's more likely to efficiently deliver the nutrients and oxygen your muscles need to power through a workout. As you lose more weight, the body changes and joints and bones that might not have experienced pressure before will suddenly start to experience intense pressure. The soreness and stiffness that go along with exercising and losing weight can be relieved by chiropractic care. Once the pain is addressed, you can keep moving forward towards your goals.

CHAPTER 25
Inset by Eric F. Watts D.C.

I have been asked a specific question numerous times in practice: Why do people still need chiropractic care, despite having a great diet, with little inflammation? Perhaps someone has changed their diet, and lost a bunch of weight and feels better than they ever have in their whole life, but they still feel the need to get adjusted every now and then. Why is that? There is an answer, and the answer is pretty simple: Life happens. Life, however, IS complicated. And those complications are not only dietary, but also (from a chiropractor's point of view) physical or structural, chemical, and emotional and even spiritual. I'm sure there are other complications as well.

We can optimize our diets, eat perfectly for ourselves every day and still have physical, and emotional challenges to our sense of wellbeing. An example of this in the physical realm could be as simple as 'level of activity'. Too little activity in the body can produce a whole set of problems; low back and hip discomfort tend to develop in an underactive person. It's as if sitting becomes a repetitive stress injury to those areas that are holding you up. Too much activity can cause pain and injury as well. These injuries of over-activity are common to weekend warrior types; sprains and strains. There are many other examples of physical and structural challenges to the body as well; just having to lift something heavy, or in an awkward way can sometimes be a problem for us.

Another example of how life might happen in such a way to challenge your ability to be in optimum shape is to experience periods of emotional stress. Almost everyone can tell you where they 'store' their stress in their body. Many people will say it's the shoulders, or the neck, or the jaw. This stored stress can end up as painful areas after a while.

Chemical stresses to the body can alter the way we adapt to our environment. Water consumption, for example, can have an effect; even being slightly dehydrated can have a large impact on skeletal muscle performance. So, if your muscles are not performing optimally, then you can expect challenges to your spine and extremities too.

Any one of the above examples can lead to a trip to your chiropractor for help. Most people experience several, or even all the above examples every single day.

Ok, fine. So, things get us stressed out, but why do things have to get out of whack in the spine? They just do. And what makes it go out? Just about everything. Let me elaborate: as chiropractors, we are trained to learn in school the 5 hallmarks of inflammation, and we learn them in Latin. They are: rubor (its red), dolor (it hurts), calor (it's hot), tumor (it's swollen), and functio lesa (it doesn't work as well). The last one is the most overlooked, and probably the most important one. Something that is inflamed just does not work as well. If that something is your spine, then your spine is not working as well. And what is the function of the spine? Just about everything. The nerves that flow through the spine control, to some extent, all the functioning of the entire body. So, it follows that now everything is not working as well.

Chiropractic care, at its core, is about having ease in the nervous system, or restoring optimal function to the nervous system. If you have an inflamed system, and EVERYTHING is not working as well, why not restore normal function? Why not exercise it properly? Why not eat well? These modalities are extremely important to the optimum functioning of your entire body, and should not be overlooked.

So my final answer to the question of why do we need chiropractic, even if we eat well is: Because life happens, and you need to do life better. Eating well helps you do life better. Reducing stress helps you do life better. Eating properly helps you do life better EVERY DAY. And chiropractic helps you do life better.

CHAPTER 26
Maintaining a Positive Attitude

If you split your time between feeling great about yourself for following your new anti-inflammatory diet and berating yourself when you mess up, you'll never get where you want to be. So, it's time to change your attitude about weight loss. Labeling all food as the enemy and talking negatively to yourself when you eat is a recipe for long-term failure. Changing how you interact with food and how you feel about your diet and exercise can seriously affect how well you stick to your healthy living plan and how well you keep the weight off. Here's how:

1. **Be careful with your words.** How you talk to yourself (either out loud or just in your head), can affect you deeply. Negative thoughts, even when you've been "bad," can drive you to do more bad behaviors. If you hate yourself, you won't want to help yourself. On the other hand, if you love yourself, you'll want only the best things, so be nice to yourself and be careful about the words you use when talking to yourself.
2. **Don't starve yourself.** The problem with a restrictive food diet is that it can feel extremely uncomfortable. The thought of eating just what's allowed in that diet and nothing else for the rest of your life is devastating. Instead, focus on changing your entire relationship with food. Think of it as fuel—you only want to put the best fuel in your body, right?
3. **Discover the difference in physical versus emotional hunger.** We all sometimes mistake emotional hunger for physical hunger. It's time for you to stop and take a moment when you're feeling hungry to look inward and ask yourself which type of hunger you're feeling now. Don't let emotional triggers

dictate when you eat. Find another way to curb those hungers, and only eat when you are physically hungry.
4. **Don't let social situations always be eating situations.** Too often, food and being social are interconnected. Your friends want to go to a restaurant to catch up. You got a promotion so your husband takes you out to dinner. This creates correlation between food and fun that can cause you, at least subconsciously, to believe that food is synonymous with fun.
5. **Be realistic and take your time.** *The Biggest Loser* isn't reality. Those people work out eight hours a day and eat highly regimented meals (and sometimes they still gain weight). One to two pounds of weight loss a week is reasonable. Ten pounds a week is not.

CHAPTER 27
10 Ways to Achieve Lasting Happiness

Few people believe that they have achieved maximum happiness and most people want to be happier in their everyday lives. Sadness can come from any facet of life, from career, to health, to even just the way we think about ourselves. Here are ten ways to achieve real and lasting happiness.

1. **Get to know yourself.** Most people assume they are more fearful, cautious, and unworthy than they are. Why? Because they don't know themselves. You don't know what you're made of until you get out and test your limits.
2. **Learn to be honest.** People let sadness and anger build up, instead of being honest about how they feel. This stored resentment can lead to a lot of unhappiness. Learning to be 100% honest with ourselves and others can make life much easier.
3. **Take care of yourself.** Most people put others and their needs ahead of their own needs. While living that way is perfectly fine, you need to give yourself some time each day, just to take care of yourself.
4. **Learn how to breathe away stress and anger.** You are in control of your body and how you feel. Rhythmic breathing is the best way to get yourself to take a mental step back and process your emotions.
5. **Practice patience.** Patience is one of the most difficult characteristics to cultivate, and it only happens through concerted effort.
6. **Practice gratitude.** Grateful people are happy people. Like patience, it takes some time and effort to develop, just like any other skill.
7. **Serve others.** Even just saying "Hello," to someone can be a service. Actively try to brighten other's days.

8. **Learn to forgive and forget.** Holding on to ancient grudges does nothing but make you sad and sick. The saying goes, "It's like drinking poison and expecting the other person to die."
9. **Stop making excuses.** As humans, we'll dredge up an excuse not to do something. Stop letting those excuses hold you back from doing what you truly want to do.
10. **Take a risk.** This is a good way to get to know yourself and test your boundaries. Taking a big risk means there is the potential of a big reward. Developing a risk-taking spirit may sound frightening, but it can make you far happier than not taking risks.

CHAPTER 28
Raising an Anti-Inflammatory Family in an "Inflammatory" World

So, few people put real thought into what they feed their families. Everyone is so busy, and fast food and junk food seem to be so much easier and cheaper than eating healthy, whole foods. This means that most people are plagued by inflammation. Personally, our family's food expenses have declined significantly since we all started eating the anti-inflammatory diet. The reason is because we eat out less, and whole foods are less expensive than processed foods.

While it might not show its devastating effects for years, inflammation is one of the leading causes of some of the most debilitating diseases in our society, including cancer, heart disease, obesity, asthma, arthritis, irritable bowel syndrome, and many others.

Therefore, learning how to raise an anti-inflammatory family in an inflammatory world is so important. Making the change can seem difficult, especially with young children in school who will see their friends eating candy and other sugar-filled treats daily. Few schools offer healthy vegetarian or vegan options as a part of their lunch program, and give children misleading information about the "health" benefits of eating meat and drinking milk. Two items that can have inflammatory effects on most people.

The dairy industry is huge in Wisconsin where I grew up and every day in elementary school we had required breaks where we all stopped what we were doing to drink milk. Now I'm sure this was a well-intentioned program to try to provide all children with nutrition, but these days the milk is not organic or hormone-free and drinking it is not a healthy choice for young children. The free lunch program at my son's daycare first is not organic or GMO-free and includes processed "cheese" and crackers,

Cheerios, lunch meats, and other extremely inflammatory foods. We need to set our children up for a long and healthy life by teaching them healthy eating habits from the time they're eating their first foods through early adolescence and the teen years. One of the very best things you can do as a parent is model good eating behavior.

When you first embark on this journey, it may seem that eating an anti-inflammatory diet is limiting, but the truth is you will discover a whole new world of fresh foods and flavors you've been missing. Once you start ignoring items with high fructose corn syrup and sugar and chemical preservatives, you'll start trying new delicious things. You'll also start to feel great after you eat. No more will you be sluggish, exhausted or angry after meals. Your body and mind will be rejuvenated.

The reason you feel so tired after meals you currently eat is because the corporate food industry needs food to be shelf stable for months, but that makes it less healthy to eat and the processing of natural food turns it into toxic sludge for your body. There's a big difference between pickles and kimchi that are naturally preserved, just by how they're made, and bread that is laced with artificial preservatives to keep it from getting moldy as it sits on a grocery shelf for weeks. Think about this, if the microorganisms that are mold don't want to eat something, do you want to eat it? If they don't think its food after two or three weeks, then it probably isn't food.

The fact is that if you want to raise an anti-inflammatory family in a world that is teeming with inflammatory foods, you must be diligent. Right now, it may be exhausting to think about packing a healthy, anti-inflammatory lunch every day for the kids, or to find recipes for meals that don't include at least one bad-for-you ingredient. Especially if one or more of your family members is resistant to the change (and it *is* very difficult to watch your friends eat something that you can't have), getting it right, all the time, is tiring. But, you owe it to yourself and the people you feed to set everyone up for a long and healthy future. What they say is true, you don't have anything if you don't have your health!

Luckily, there are a lot of good online resources and even apps that make it possible to stick to an anti-inflammatory diet (in addition to the recipes in this book), whether you are making the change to deal with a physical condition, or just because you know it can prevent some of the most common chronic diseases a person can develop. Knowledge is power, so equip yourself and your family with as much knowledge as possible! I've included a lot of recipes at the end of this book to get you started, but with a little searching you can find an unlimited variety online as well.

Based on love, the desire to help you achieve wellness, and the knowledge gained from my own research, I set my goal here to compile a book that would be both informational and motivational. If I help only one person change their life for the better, then I've done my job.

I hope you have found in this book information that will help you to evaluate your daily eating habits and determine what you need to change in your life. It's a process, so go slow and remain positive and you will heal yourself with food. As I set out to write the book I found myself focusing on my own daily eating habits, and I found areas that I too still need to work on. I hope the knowledge you gain will change your life as it has changed mine.

CHAPTER 29
Animals and Inflammation: Why Anti-Inflammatory Should Also be Vegetarian or Vegan

> "G-d did not permit Adam and his wife to kill a creature and to eat its flesh. Only every green herb shall they all eat together."
> — MAIMONIDES

The purpose of the Vitality anti-inflammatory diet is to lessen the inflammatory response in the human body, and eating a responsible vegetarian diet is a way to lessen our impact on other living creatures and on the living systems of planet Earth. So, this is a diet that is good for both people and planet.

Almost all discussion of the traditional anti-inflammatory diet includes eating animals - salmon, chicken, beef, fish, etc. But I've written this book out of respect for all life, not just my own. Eating meat perpetuates a system of massive industrial violence, pollution and extinction. Both scientists and nutritionists have judged eating meat to be unnecessary and mostly unhealthy. Therefore, to choose to be a part of this system indicates a disregard for the health of the planet, our fellow sentient beings both human animals and other creatures we love, and this in effect pollutes not only our bodies but also contaminates our moral character. A meatless diet is a worthy endeavor for a person who values compassion, humility, and integrity.

Why We Don't Eat Fish in the Vitality Anti-Inflammatory Diet

It is a mistake to think of fish just as a source of food. That is like thinking of sunlight just as a source of warmth for humans. Fish are an integral part of their ecosystem and when we remove them from that ecosystem we create a weak link in their own food chain and in the ecosystem in which they live. Because of how we fish industrially, we also do great damage, especially to barrier reefs, which are home to thousands of species of not just fish, but a wide variety of plants and animals. We often do far more damage than just removing one stage of a food chain.

Consider this question: Is eating fish more important to you than restoring our dying oceans and aqua systems? Today's fish are caught using industrial methods that our ancestors did not have access to. We don't just send out individual fishing boats. Instead, we send out mega boats with advanced sonar to fish giant portions of our waters, causing serious damage to the ocean. These "modern" techniques make it possible to get more fish in a shorter amount of time, but also cause far more damage than traditional methods would have done. We're stripping the ocean of its resources faster than it can replenish them. The huge nets and bottom trawls fisheries use now are horribly damaging. The metal nets scrape the ground and pull up everything. It's not just the fish, it's the coral that is destroyed during fishing and the other ocean creatures that are harmed. Eating fish, for most people, is not a necessity. While many people who live near water will find that fish is often a part of local menus and that fresh fish is easier to find there than farther inland, it is not their only option. Those who believe that fish are meant to be eaten by humans perpetuate overfishing in lakes, streams, rivers, and in the ocean, seriously damaging fragile ecosystems. Instead of harvesting fish species to extinction, we should be protecting them - not just to protect the fish and the vital water systems on our planet - but to protect ourselves, too. The methods by which fish are raised or caught in the wild are completely destructive to the planet. It is always a choice whether you eat fish.

Fish must consume thousands of plants during their lives to survive, and along with those plants, they consume many toxins from chemicals that have been dumped or spilled into the water supply. When you eat fish, you also eat those toxins, which can take years to be removed from your body. It's simply impossible to get fish today that haven't been contaminated by toxins or fished using unethical methods. Worst of all, most of what's pulled up from the ocean by fisheries is just dumped back into the ocean, so the death and destruction are done for nothing.

In the Vitality diet, eliminating fish from the diet just makes sense, not only because of how fishing impacts the planet, but also because of how eating fish impacts the body. Part of eating responsibly and mindfully is knowing what is happening to the food you eat before it arrives on your table. The energy that the world needs in order to grow a plant is much less than it takes to grow a plant-eater. When we eat fish (or any animal for that matter) we are jumping ahead in the natural food chain, especially because many of the other types of meat that we raise are forced to eat fish, which is far outside of their natural diet. For example, fish is often ground up and fed to pigs and chickens.

People who eat fish regularly have a much higher concentration of mercury in their systems than people who do not eat fish, so high that it contributes to many serious conditions. People who eat carnivorous fish, such as halibut or tuna, have much higher mercury concentrations than people who do not eat fish or who eat plant-eating fish. As fish eat fish, their mercury content increases, and when we eat fish that are high on the oceanic food chain, you get a much higher dosage of mercury.

Fish accumulate toxins as they grow and the older the fish is, the more toxins it contains. And unlike cows, pigs, and chickens that are slaughtered early in life, rather than later in life, some fish are allowed to grow and develop for decades before they are harvested. This means they are far more likely to have high levels of toxins in their system.

Even fish that are raised on fish farms are not immune to this toxin-collection process. There are very few closed-system fisheries where water is recycled, nutrition is added, and the nutrients that the fish produce are saved and used. Most fisheries prefer to pen in their fish, even if they are still in the ocean. These sorts of solutions are still focused on raising fish for a capitalist market, not on raising healthy fish that will nourish people. The mass-market culture that has invaded the fishing industry makes it much more likely that a fishery is raising huge number of fish using unethical means. The only sustainable aquaculture environment is a closed one - like an aquarium. On one side, there are fish and on the other side, plants, and all have plenty of sunlight, and everything is recycled.

Today, however, the focus is not on recycling or using natural resources, but on getting the largest number of fish in stores as quickly and cheaply as possible. Our ability to kill a large number of fish in a very short amount of time far outstrips the ocean's ability to replenish the fish population or to repair the physical damage done by today's modern fishing techniques. Corporations will not stop until the last fish has been pulled from the ocean.

Eating fish is very, very rarely a true necessity. There are few situations in which there are no other choices. The main reason people eat fish in traditional anti-inflammatory diets is because they are told that fish are healthy. Well, eating fish is not healthy for you or the planet. The truth is that a plant-based diet is only limited by your imagination. There are over 250,000 different kinds of plants grown on our planet.

Fish, like everything else in this world, should not be thought of as one big mass, and especially not as just one big mass of something we can eat. They are individuals and we should value them for their individual and very necessary contribution to our world's ecosystem and continued existence.

What to consider when eating eggs

The Vitality diet strives to be cruelty free, but some recipes do include eggs. Often chickens are treated horribly and their lives are commodified like every other creature on the planet. Using marketing tactics, we are led to believe that certain labels offer improved standards for the treatment of the hens, the truth is, there's not much difference at all.

Per the Humane Society, "the truth is that the majority of egg labels have little relevance to animal welfare or, if they do, they have no official standards or any mechanism to enforce them."

If you're confused about the best choice for your health and the welfare of the hens involved, you should keep your own chickens in the backyard or buy from farmers you know that have Animal Welfare Approved farms. But, sadly almost all chickens that lay eggs will end up in the meat industry and the baby male chicks ground up for being "useless". A vegan diet is best. Here is a guide to egg labels:

Cage-Free:

- Uncaged, inside barns.
- Generally, no access to outdoors.
- Can engage in many of their natural behaviors such as walking, nesting, and spreading their wings.
- Beak cutting and forced molting through starvation are permitted.

Free-Range:

- Uncaged inside barns.
- Have some access to outdoors, but there are no restrictions regarding what they can be fed, and no requirements for the amount, duration or quality of outdoor access.
- Because they are not caged, they can engage in many natural behaviors such as nesting and foraging.
- Beak cutting and forced molting through starvation are permitted.

Pasture-Raised:

- Pasture-raised hens are kept outdoors for most of the year, on a pasture covered with living plants, and are kept indoors at night for protection.

- However, because there is no regulation of the term, there are no restrictions regarding what the birds can be fed and no requirements for the amount of time spent on the pasture, the amount of space per bird, or the quality of the pasture.
- Beak cutting and forced molting through starvation are permitted.

Certified Organic:

- The same standards as Free-Range, with the only differences being that they are fed an organic, all-vegetarian diet free of antibiotics and pesticides, as required by the U.S. Department of Agriculture's National Organic Program and compliance is verified through third-party auditing.
- Still permits cruel and inhumane factory farm practices such as the space per bird less than a sheet of paper, battery cages, kept indoors always and only little considering for perching and nesting requirements when the eggs are 'cage-free'.

Animal Welfare Approved means:

- The birds are cage-free with at least 1.8 square feet (259 square inches) of floor space provided per bird, and they must be able to perform natural behaviors such as nesting, perching and dust-bathing.
- Hens must also be provided continuous access to an outdoor area for ranging and foraging. This outdoor area must be covered with growing vegetation and must provide at least 4 square feet (576 square inches) per bird.
- There are requirements for stocking density, perching and nesting boxes.
- Forced molting through starvation and beak cutting are prohibited, as is feed containing meat or animal byproducts.

While the USDA has defined the meaning of "free-range" for some poultry products, there are no government-regulated standards in "free-range" or "pasture-raised" egg production required to make the claim. For all of the above terms, there is also no mandatory third-party auditing. So whether or not the standards are followed depends on each individual farm and their standards.

The best way to know for sure how the hens are treated is to visit the farm and see for yourself. Source your eggs from local, ethical farmers with plenty of space for the hens to roam and thrive. Quiz your local farmer on their practices - that way you know exactly how they are treated, and you'll be able to see and taste the difference in the quality of the eggs.

Or if you'd prefer not to eat eggs, check out the egg substitute chart below.

1 EGG EQUALS	USE	NOTES
1/2 banana, mashed	Pancakes, cakes, breads	Very ripe bananas will add sweetness
1/4 cup applesauce or 1/4 cup ripe mashed pears	Breads, cakes, brownies	Avoid using more than 1/4 cup total in any recipe
1/4 cup natural or Greek Yogurt	Brownies, smoothies	Can cause final product to be heavier
2.5 tablespoons ground flax mixed with the 3 tablespoons water, set in fridge for 10 minutes	Granola bars, smoothies	Adds earthy, nutty taste and chewy texture
1 tablespoon coconut oil mixed with 2 tablespoons baking powder & 2 teaspoons water	Gluten free cooking	Adds earthy, nutty taste and chewy texture
1 tablespoon chia seeds mixed with 3 tablespoons water, set in fridge for 10 minutes.	Smoothies, baked goods	Adds fats to the recipe, can be tricky to work with
1/4 cup pureed prunes (or any high pectin fruit)	Breads, cakes, brownies	Binds and thickens
1/4 cup pumpkin, mashed (canned worked well, choose BPA free cans)	Breads, brownies	Adds sweetness to the recipe
1/4 cup potato, cooked and mashed (sweet potato might be yummy)	Savory dishes	Can be heavy
1 tablespoon agar with 1 tablespoon water, whipped and chilled	Gluten free cooking	Used to replace egg whites only

Part 4: Anti-Inflammatory Meal Ideas

CHAPTER 1
Breakfast

When you hear cartoon characters on Saturday morning kids' show say that "breakfast is the most important meal of the day," or are reminded of that adage by a parent, friend, or coworker who discovered you've skipped that meal, it can start to sound cliché. The reality is, however, that no matter how many times you've been nagged about eating breakfast, breakfast really *is* the most important meal of the day and there's the science to prove it.

Most people skip breakfast for one of two reasons: either they are too busy in the morning and just can't find the time even for a bowl of quick oats, or they actively choose not to eat breakfast, believing they are saving calories that they can then eat later in the day. Neither of these are good reasons to skip breakfast. No matter why you skip it, your body is going to be starving by mid-morning if you skip this meal because you haven't eaten for over eight hours, and you'll be putting it off another four hours if you decide not to eat breakfast.

Breakfast is the foundation of weight loss and maintaining weight loss. People who are consistent breakfast eaters not only lose more weight, but they also keep it off for longer than those who did not eat breakfast. This is especially true for people who lose a great deal of weight. You must eat breakfast to maintain your weight loss.

One study found that young girls, between the ages of nine and nineteen who ate breakfast, were less likely to be overweight in their developmental years than girls that didn't. Why does this happen? Because people who skip breakfast not only feel ravenous by the next meal (which promotes overeating), they often reward themselves for "skipping" a meal (and "saving" calories), by snacking, or eating higher calorie foods over the course of a day.

What kind of breakfast you eat matters, too. Those who ate healthier breakfasts, like oatmeal and avocado, ate healthier throughout the day, while those that loaded up on trans-fat and sugar in the morning, would often continue to eat that way throughout the day.

In the United States, sugary, meat heavy, breakfasts are the go-to choice for many. This is a relic of a time long ago where farmers needed this type of meal to have enough energy until lunch. It was designed to sustain hours of manual labor with calories to spare. However, we're not a rural society anymore. Often, work consists of sitting in a relatively inactive fashion for hours at a time with only the glow of a computer monitor to keep us company. Most of us do not hold manual labor positions and have absolutely no use for high calorie meals. And even if we did, we can do a lot better than eating a ton of grease and processed foods. If you do hold a white-collar position, wouldn't the ingestion of lots of plant protein and anti-inflammatory foods serve you better? Of course, it would!

If you eat within 30 minutes of waking up, you can jumpstart your metabolism and get it rolling for the rest of the day. While asleep, our metabolism is designed to slow down and conserve energy. It's resting, in a sense, along with the rest of our body. Your job in the morning is to wake it up. You need to do this early in the day. In fact, the sooner the better. Make sure when you do this that you get enough to sustain you, but not overwhelm your body with too many calories. You want to focus on getting the perfect balance of whole grains, proteins, and good fats (omega-3 if you've got 'em handy). A simple breakfast in this regard is an avocado and seasoned black beans or organic Scottish oatmeal. You could eat these breakfasts every day.

Avoid sugar laden foods such as donuts or most cereals. They are toxic, so get into the habit of thinking of them as poison, like a piece of plastic or something else that's not food. Think about how hard your poor body must work to get that crap out of your system! If you must have something sweet, grab an apple or a handful of berries (preferably blueberries). If you can't eliminate coffee, remember to look for other alternative forms that are less toxic to your body like organic, low caffeine versions, or matcha green tea.

Your breakfast lays the foundation for your day, so make sure you eat it and make it a good one!

Breakfast Recipes

1 Vegetable Frittata

Makes 1 - 2 servings.

Organic Ingredients:

- 1 yellow bell pepper
- 1 red bell pepper
- 1 cup fresh peas
- 1 head broccoli cut into small pieces
- 6 eggs beaten
- 1/2 cup unflavored rice or soy milk
- 1 Tbsp. fresh basil chopped in ribbons
- 1 teaspoon fresh oregano chopped in ribbons
- 1/4 cup fresh cashews broken into pieces for garnish

Simple Preparation:
Place the yellow and red peppers under your oven broiler on a sheet pan for 7 minutes until they're skins are lightly charred. Place them in a bag and seal tightly so that the skins will come off easily. Then slice the peppers thinly. Reduce the heat of the oven to 400 degrees Fahrenheit. Grease a 9-inch round pan. Place the peppers, peas and broccoli pieces on the bottom of the pan to form a thin layer. Beat the eggs, milk, basil, and oregano together and pour over the vegetables. Bake in the oven for 35 minutes or until the top has turned slightly brown. Remove the frittata from the oven and let it cool. Then slice it into wedges and top with cashews.

2 Cherry Quinoa Porridge

Makes 2 servings.

Organic Ingredients:

- 1 cup filtered water
- 1/2 teaspoon of real vanilla extract
- 1/4 teaspoon of ground cinnamon
- 1/2 cup of dry quinoa
- 1/2 cup dried unsweetened or fresh cherries

Optional: you can add a tablespoon of honey if you really want, but make sure of the source and remember that we're trying to cut back the sugar. Optional: you can also add a few teaspoons of fresh slivered almonds on top, giving a nice texture and adding essential fats and oils in the process.

Simple Preparation:
Simply combine all the ingredients (excluding the optional honey and almonds) into a medium saucepan. Bring them to a boil of medium-high heat. Reduce and simmer for approximately 15 minutes, making sure that the quinoa has cooked thoroughly and is tender. Serve drizzled with the honey and/or almonds.

3 Baked Blueberry Oatmeal Breakfast Pudding

Makes 4-6 servings.

Organic Ingredients:

- 1/2 cup lightly toasted hazelnuts, with skin
- 1/2 cup lightly toasted cashews
- 1/2 cup old-fashioned rolled oats (not instant–use certified gluten-free oats for GF)
- 3/4 cup unsweetened applesauce
- 2 teaspoons pure real vanilla extract
- 2 Tbsps. agave nectar or 10 drops pure stevia liquid
- 2 teaspoons cinnamon
- 1/8 teaspoon fine sea salt
- 1-1/4 cups unsweetened, plain or vanilla soy or almond milk
- 1/2 cup fresh or frozen blueberries (do not thaw first if frozen)

Simple Preparation:
Preheat oven to 350°F. In the bowl of a high-speed blender*, place the nuts, oats, applesauce, vanilla, agave, cinnamon and salt. Pour in the milk overall and blend for about a minute, until perfectly smooth and creamy. Pour mixture into a 6 cup oven safe casserole dish, then gently fold in the blueberries (scatter a few extra blueberries over the top if you like, as they won't sink). Bake in preheated oven for 40-50 minutes, rotating the casserole about halfway through, until the edges begin to puff and crack and the top appears dry. Allow to cool somewhat before serving; may be served warm or cold. Store, covered, up to 4 days in the refrigerator. May be frozen. *To make with a regular blender: Pour in the milk first, then add the remaining ingredients (except blueberries). You may need to blend in batches to achieve an equally smooth consistency.

4 Heavenly Carrot Cake Baked Oatmeal

Makes 4 servings.

Organic Ingredients:

- 2 1/4 cups rolled oats
- 1 1/2 teaspoons ground cinnamon
- 1 1/2 teaspoons aluminum-free baking powder
- 1/4 teaspoon fine grain sea salt
- 1 1/2 cups lightly packed shredded carrots
- 2 1/2 cups unsweetened almond milk (or non-dairy milk of choice)
- 1/3 cup agave syrup
- 2 teaspoons pure vanilla extract
- 1 1/2 teaspoons freshly grated ginger (or try ½ teaspoon ground ginger)
- 1/4 cup raisins
- 1/2 cup chopped walnut halves

Simple Preparation:
Preheat oven to 375°F and lightly grease a 10-cup/2.5 qt. casserole dish. In a large bowl, mix together the rolled oats, cinnamon, baking powder, and salt. In a medium bowl, whisk together the wet ingredients: shredded carrot, almond milk, agave syrup, vanilla, and fresh ginger. Add the wet mixture to dry mixture and stir until combined. Pour mixture into prepared dish and smooth out with a spoon. Press down on the oatmeal with a spoon (or your hands) so the oats sink into the milk. Sprinkle on the walnuts and raisins and press down lightly again. Bake, uncovered, for 35 minutes until lightly golden along edge. The oatmeal will still look a bit soft or wet in some spots when it comes out of the oven, but it will firm up as it cools. Let cool for about 10 minutes before serving. When the baked oatmeal is fully cool, it will firm up enough to be sliced into squares. Enjoy it warm, at room temp, or chilled straight from the fridge.

5 Cinnamon Raisin Oatmeal Oat Cake

Makes 4 servings.

Organic Ingredients:

- 1/2 cup organic cold-pressed coconut oil, measured in liquid form
- 1/4 cup agave nectar
- 1 1/2 cups coconut milk
- 2 organic eggs
- 2 teaspoons real vanilla
- 3 cups certified gluten-free rolled oats
- 1/2 teaspoon sea salt
- 1 Tbsp. arrowroot powder
- 1 teaspoon ground cinnamon
- 1 Tbsp. ground chia seeds (or flax meal)
- 1/2 cup golden, or dark, raisins or apple pieces

Topping:

- 2 Tbsps. toasted almond slivers
- 2 teaspoons ground chia seeds (or flax meal)
- 1/2 teaspoon ground cinnamon

Simple Preparation:
In medium bowl, using stand or hand mixer, mix together: Coconut oil and agave nectar until well blended. Add milk, eggs, and vanilla. In separate large bowl, sift together: gluten-free oats, sea salt, baking powder, cinnamon, and ground chia (or flax) seed. Mix with the mixer on low speed: gently add in dry mixture and mix for 1 minute until blended. Then fold in raisins (or apples). Then pour mixture into a non-toxic non-stick 8×8 baking dish. Cover with plastic wrap and refrigerate overnight. In small bowl mix together topping ingredients and set aside until morning. In morning: preheat oven to 350°F. Set assembled dish on your counter to bring to room temp (about 20 minutes). Sprinkle topping mixture evenly over cake and bake for about 25 minutes, or until feels slightly firm to touch. Top with ground cinnamon, or eat just as is.

6 Date-Orange Breakfast Spread

Eat this as a topping on quinoa, brown rice or barley.

Makes 2 servings.

Organic Ingredients:

- 1 cup finely chopped pitted dates (about 1/2 pound)
- 1 Tbsp. finely grated orange rind
- 2 Tbsps. fresh orange juice
- 1/2 teaspoon ground cinnamon
- 1/8 teaspoon sea salt

Simple Preparation:
Combine all ingredients, stirring until blended. Chill 30 minutes.

7 Blissful Blueberry Banana Spelt Muffins

Makes 12 servings.

Organic Ingredients:

- 3/4 cup mashed ripe banana (about 2 medium)
- 3/4 cup + 2 tablespoons unsweetened almond milk
- 1 teaspoon apple cider vinegar
- 1/4 cup agave syrup
- 1 teaspoon pure vanilla extract
- 1/4 cup coconut oil, melted
- 2 cups light spelt flour
- 2 teaspoons baking powder
- 1.5 teaspoons cinnamon
- 1/2 tsp fine grain sea salt
- 1/2 tsp baking soda
- 1/2 cup chopped walnut pieces
- 1 cup frozen or fresh blueberries (see note)

Simple Preparation:
Preheat oven to 350°F and grease a muffin tin. In a medium bowl, mash bananas and measure out 3/4 cup. If you have any leftover mashed banana you can freeze it for a smoothie. Place mashed banana into medium bowl along with the milk, vinegar, agave syrup, and vanilla. No need to stir it yet. Melt the coconut oil in a small pot over low heat. Set aside. In a large bowl, mix together the dry ingredients (flour, baking powder, cinnamon, salt, and baking soda). Stir coconut oil into the wet mixture. Pour wet ingredients onto the dry ingredients and stir until just combined. Do not overmix as spelt is a fragile little flour. Gently fold in the walnuts and then the blueberries, being sure not to overmix as this can result in dense muffins. Spoon about a heaping 1/4 cup of batter into each muffin tin, filling each tin about 3/4 full (they will seem very full, but this is normal!) I like to press a few extra blueberries on top of each so they look pretty after baking. Bake at 350F for 25 minutes until a toothpick comes out clean. Cool in pan for 5-8 minutes and then transfer muffins to a cooling rack and cool for another 15 minutes.

8 Bircher Muesli

Makes 1 serving.

Organic Ingredients:

- 1/2 cup oats
- 2 Tbsps. chia seeds
- 1 Tbsp. pumpkin seeds
- 1 1/2 cups almond or coconut milk
- 1 Tbsp. agave nectar
- 1/2 teaspoon of all-natural vanilla extract
- 1 teaspoon lemon juice
- 2 ripe pears
- 1 pinch of ground cinnamon
- 1/4 cup dried sour cherries or cranberries

Simple Preparation:
The night before, put the oats, chia seeds and pumpkin seeds into a bowl or container, pour over the milk, and add the agave nectar, vanilla and lemon juice. Mix well, then cover and pop into the fridge overnight. In the morning, chop the pears into little chunks, sprinkle over the cinnamon and add the sour cherries and either layer them up with the oats and seeds in a glass or bowl, or if you're in a hurry just run out of the door with everything in a little container.

9 Eggless Vegan Omelets

Makes 1 - 2 servings.

Organic Ingredients:
Omelet:

- 5 oz (3/4 cup) firm silken tofu, drained and gently patted dry
- 2 Tbsps. hummus (see below)
- 2 large cloves garlic, minced
- 2 Tbsps. nutritional yeast
- Salt and black pepper
- 1/4 teaspoon paprika
- 1 teaspoon arrowroot powder

Filling:

- 1 heaping cup veggies of choice (I like onion, asparagus, mushrooms, spinach)

Simple Preparation:
Preheat oven to 375°F. Prep veggies, drain and dry tofu, and minced garlic. Set aside. Heat a small-to-medium, oven-safe skillet over medium heat. Once hot, add olive oil and minced garlic and cook for 1-2 minutes or until just lightly golden brown. Transfer garlic to food processor, along with remaining omelet ingredients (tofu and arrowroot powder) and mix to combine, scraping down sides as needed. Add just a touch of water to thin – 1-2 Tbsps. at most. Set aside. To the still warm skillet over medium heat, add a bit more olive oil and the veggies. Season with salt and pepper and sauté to desired doneness. I like to start with onions and tomatoes, then add mushrooms, and end with spinach so each has proper time to cook. Set aside. Remove skillet from heat and make sure it's coated with enough oil so the omelet doesn't stick. Add back 1/4 of the veggies and spoon on the omelet batter, spreading it gently with a spoon or rubber spatula, being careful not to tear or cause gaps. The thinner and more evenly you can spread it the better. So you may not end up using it all. Cook over medium heat on the stovetop for 5 minutes until the edges start to dry. Then place in 375 degree oven and bake until dry and deep golden brown – 10-15 minutes. The longer it bakes the less soft/wet it will be, so if you prefer a more well

done omelet, cook closer to 15 or more. Using an oven mitt, in the last few minutes of cooking carefully add remaining veggies back on top of the omelet and cook another 1-2 minutes to warm through. Carefully remove from oven with oven mitt and fold over gently with a spatula.

10 Mushroom and Onion Omelet

Makes 1 serving.

Organic Ingredients:

- 2 Tbsps. olive oil
- 3 eggs, beaten
- 3 Tbsps. unsweetened coconut milk
- 1/4 cup mushroom, sliced
- 1/8 teaspoon freshly ground black pepper
- 3 Tbsps. white onions, diced

Optional toppings: chopped cilantro, chives or parsley

Simple Preparation:
Heat olive oil in a frying pan. Beat together the eggs, coconut milk and black pepper until frothy. Cook the mushrooms and onions in a pan over medium high heat until they start to brown. Remove the vegetables from the pan. Then add the egg mixture to the pan and cook until almost set, until you can flip it over without it falling apart, cook on the other side until set. Top 1/2 of the omelet with the cooked mushrooms and onions and fold over. You can add a little freshness by topping the omelet with cilantro, chives or parsley.

11 Ginger Protein Pancakes

Makes 4 small pancakes.

Organic Ingredients:

- 2/3 cup almond milk
- 1/4 cup egg whites or 1 flax egg (1 tablespoon freshly ground flax + 3 tablespoon water)
- 1 Tbsp. agave nectar
- 1 Tbsp. chia seeds
- 1 teaspoon pure vanilla extract
- 10 drops vanilla stevia
- 2/3 cup chickpea flour
- 1 teaspoon gluten-free baking powder
- 1 teaspoon ground cinnamon
- 1 teaspoon ground ginger
- 1/8 teaspoon ground cloves

Simple Preparation:
Combine the almond milk and chia seeds and allow to sit for 10 minutes – this will get the chia all gelatinous and good for your digestion. Alternatively, allow the chia to soak overnight in the milk, then add to the recipe. Preheat a small non-toxic non-stick pan on medium-low heat for 2 minutes. Meanwhile, combine the dry ingredients in a separate bowl, then add to the wet ingredients. Stir until just mixed. Pour 1/4 of the mixture into the preheated pan. Allow the first side to cook for 3-4 minutes, or until bubbles form and the edges begin to turn golden. Flip and allow to cook for another 1-2 minutes. Place completed pancake on cooling rack and repeat with remaining batter. Serve with chopped apples.

12 Strawberry Shortcake Stacked Pancakes

Makes 8 small pancakes.

Organic Ingredients:

- 1 cup + 1/4 cup almond flour
- 1/2 cup shredded, unsweetened coconut
- 1 teaspoon baking powder
- 1/4 teaspoon baking soda
- generous 1/4 teaspoon nutmeg
- generous 1/4 teaspoon allspice
- 1/4 teaspoon cinnamon
- Pinch or two kosher salt
- 3/4 cup coconut milk
- 1/2 teaspoon pure vanilla extract
- 1 Tbsp. pure agave syrup
- 3/4 cup warm water
- olive oil, for the skillet
- Strawberry Banana Soft Serve (3 strawberries + 1 frozen banana, processed in food processor)

Simple Preparation:

Preheat oven to 250°F and grab a baking sheet. Whisk the dry ingredients (almond flour, coconut, baking soda, baking powder, spices, and salt) in a medium sized bowl. In a small bowl, whisk together the wet ingredients (coconut milk, warm water, vanilla, agave syrup) and then add to the dry ingredients. Whisk well until no clumps remain. Preheat the skillet over medium heat and add some oil on the pan. Pour 1/4 cup of batter, per pancake, onto the skillet and quickly smooth out a circle with the back of a spoon. Cook until small bubbles appear on the surface and the bottoms of pancakes are golden. Reduce heat if necessary. Transfer to baking sheet and place in the oven to keep warm. Meanwhile, slice about 20 strawberries. Stack the pancakes and top with the strawberry banana soft serve. Drizzle with agave syrup and serve immediately.

13 Coconut Pancakes

Makes 4 pancakes.

Organic Ingredients:

- 6 Tbsps. unsweetened plain or vanilla almond milk
- 2 Tbsps. finely ground flax seeds
- 1 Tbsp. extra virgin olive oil
- 1 teaspoon apple cider vinegar
- 6-8 drops plain or vanilla stevia liquid, to your taste
- 1 teaspoon pure vanilla extract
- 1/3 cup unsweetened shredded toasted coconut
- 2 Tbsps. brown rice flour
- 1 Tbsp. coconut flour
- 1 teaspoon baking powder
- 1/2 teaspoon baking soda
- 1 egg white
- 1/8 teaspoon fine sea salt

Simple Preparation:
In the bottom of a medium bowl, whisk together the milk, egg white, flax seeds, oil, vinegar, stevia and vanilla. Stir in the coconut to coat. Into the same bowl, sift the brown rice flour, coconut flour, baking powder, baking soda, and salt. Stir quickly to blend; do not over mix. It will be thick. Heat a large nonstick frying pan over medium-low heat (cooking over slightly lower heat, but for a longer time, ensures that the pancakes are fully cooked). Using a large ice cream scoop or spatula, scoop about 1/4 of the batter into the pan and spread it fairly thin with the back of a spoon or spatula (it should be too thick to spread on its own). Allow to cook for 4-6 minutes, until the edges of the pancakes begin to dry and the bottoms are a very deep golden brown. Flip and cook another 4-5 minutes, until fully cooked. You want the pancakes to be very well browned. Serve with almond butter, fresh fruit topping, or any other topping of your choice. May be frozen.

14 Almonds and Berries Bowl

Makes 1 serving.

Organic Ingredients:

- 1 Gala or Fuji apple, diced
- 1/2 cup fresh or frozen mixed berries
- 2 Tbsps. raw almonds, broken
- 1 Tbsp. raw pumpkin seeds
- 1/2 cup unsweetened almond milk

Simple Preparation:
Pour almond milk over apples, nuts and berries in bowl.

15 Almond Butter Banana Chocolate Chip Breakfast Bowl

Makes 1 serving.

Organic Ingredients:

- 1 banana
- 1 egg white
- 1 teaspoon real vanilla extract
- 1/3 cup old fashioned oats
- 1/4 teaspoon baking powder
- 1 Tbsp. very dark sugar free chocolate chips or carob chips
- 1/4 teaspoon cinnamon
- 1 Tbsp. creamy almond butter

Simple Preparation:

In a microwavable cereal bowl, mash the banana with a fork and mix in the egg. Whip it well. Stir in the real vanilla extract. Add the oats, baking powder and dash of cinnamon. Stir until fully incorporated. Stir in the very dark chocolate chips. Microwave for 1 minute, 45 seconds. Spread the almond butter on top and enjoy while warm.

16 Beet Breakfast Bowl

Makes 1 serving.

Organic Ingredients:

- 1 cup cooked leftover grains (quinoa, brown rice, millet, etc.)
- 1 small beet, finely grated (be sure it's fine—it will meld better with the other ingredients)
- 1 Tbsp. raw or lightly toasted sunflower or pumpkin seeds, or coarsely chopped walnuts, or almonds
- 1 Tbsp. chia seeds
- 1 cup unsweetened plain or vanilla almond, soy, rice or hemp milk
- 1 teaspoon cinnamon sprinkling hemp seeds, if desired handful goji berries, raisins, chopped dates, etc.
- Add the milk of your choice when serving.

Simple Preparation:
Place all ingredients in a bowl, mix, and enjoy with a splash of your favorite milk. Makes one serving. Best eaten immediately.

17 Multi-Grain Good Morning Bars

Makes 12 bars.

Organic Ingredients:

- 2 Tbsps. ground flax seeds
- 6 Tbsps. filtered water
- 1/2 cup quinoa flakes
- 1/2 cup millet flakes
- 1 cup rolled oats
- 1/2 cup oat flour
- 1/2 cup oat bran
- 1 teaspoon cinnamon
- 1 Tbsp. orange zest
- 1 Tbsp. lemon zest
- 3 Tbsps. agave nectar
- 1 teaspoon real vanilla extract
- 1 cup unsweetened applesauce
- 1/2 cup dried apricots, chopped
- 1/2 cup unsweetened shredded coconut
- 1/2 cup macadamia nuts, chopped

Simple Preparation:
Pre-heat oven to 350°F degrees. Line an 11 x 7 baking dish with parchment paper. Mix ground flax seeds and water together and let sit. In a large bowl mix together quinoa, millet and oat flakes. Stir in the oat flour, bran, cinnamon and zests. Add the agave nectar, vanilla extract, and apple sauce and flax/water mixture. Mix until well combined. Fold in the dried apricots, shredded coconut and macadamia nuts. Transfer the mixture into the lined baking dish, spreading it evenly and smoothing the top. Bake for 25 minutes, or until the edges brown slightly. Let cool completely before cutting. These bars will stay good for a few days in an airtight container. They also freeze well for later enjoyment.

18 Fruit and Nut Breakfast Treats

Makes 12 servings.

Organic Ingredients:

- 1/2 cup raw walnuts, chopped
- 1/2 cup raw pecans, chopped
- 1/2 cup raw sunflower seeds
- 1/2 cup raisins
- 2 Tbsps. coconut flour
- 2 teaspoons ground cinnamon
- 1/4 teaspoon sea salt
- 1 medium very ripe banana, mashed well
- 2 Tbsps. unsweetened applesauce
- 2 Tbsps. ground flaxseed
- 1 Tbsp. grapeseed oil or melted coconut oil
- 1 Tbsp. agave syrup

Simple Preparation:

Preheat the oven to 350°F. Line 12 cups of a standard muffin pan with paper liners. In a large mixing bowl, combine the walnuts, pecans, sunflower seeds, raisins, coconut flour, cinnamon, and salt. In a separate bowl, whisk the mashed banana, applesauce, flaxseed, oil, and agave syrup. Stir the wet ingredients into the nut mixture to combine thoroughly. Divide the mixture evenly among the lined muffin cups. Using your fingers, press the mixture firmly into the bottom of each cup. Bake for 20 minutes or until lightly browned and just firm to the touch. Cool completely. Remove paper liners and serve. (Store in an airtight container in the refrigerator.)

19 Grain Free Microwave English Muffin

Makes one muffin.

Organic Ingredients:

- 1 1/2 tablespoons almond flour
- 2 Tbsps. coconut flour
- 1 teaspoon olive oil
- 1 egg
- pinch of salt
- 1/4 teaspoon baking powder
- 2 Tbsps. water

Simple Preparation:
Mix all ingredients together in small bowl. Pour in separate microwave safe bowl sprayed with nonstick spray. Microwave for 2 – 2 1/2 minutes.

20 Vegetable Frittata

Makes 6 servings.

Organic Ingredients:

- 1 small zucchini, 1-inch-diced
- 1 green bell pepper, seeded and 1 1/2-inch-diced
- 1 yellow bell pepper, seeded and 1 1/2-inch-diced
- 1 red onion, 1 1/2-inch-diced
- 1/3 cup olive oil
- Kosher salt and freshly ground black pepper
- 2 teaspoons minced garlic (2 cloves)
- 12 extra-large eggs
- 1 cup unsweetened rice milk or soy milk
- 1/3 cup chopped scallions, white and green parts (3 scallions)

Simple Preparation:
Preheat the oven to 425°F degrees. Place the zucchini, peppers, and onion on a sheet pan. Drizzle with the olive oil, sprinkle with 1 1/2 teaspoons salt and 1/2 teaspoon pepper, and toss well. Bake for 15 minutes. Add the garlic, toss again, and bake for another 15 minutes. Remove from the oven and turn the oven to 350 degrees. Meanwhile, in a large bowl, whisk together the eggs, milk, 1 teaspoon salt, and 1/2 teaspoon pepper. In a 10-inch ovenproof sauté pan, sauté the scallions with a tiny bit of olive oil over medium-low heat for 1 minute. Add the roasted vegetables to the pan and toss with the scallions. Pour the egg mixture over the vegetables and cook for 2 minutes over medium-low heat without stirring. Transfer the pan to the oven and bake the frittata for 20 to 30 minutes, until puffed and set in the middle. Cut into 6 or 8 wedges and serve hot.

21 Spicy Breakfast Scrambled Eggs

Makes 2 servings.

Organic Ingredients:

- 4 beaten eggs
- 1 Tbsp. olive oil
- 1/2 onion, chopped
- 1 green bell pepper, chopped
- 1 lb package very firm sprouted tofu crumbled
- 1/2 cup cilantro, chopped
- 1/2 jalapeno, deseeded and minced
- 1 avocado

Simple Preparation:

In a large skillet, sauté onion in olive oil over medium-high heat for 2-3 minutes. Add green pepper and cook for another 2-3 minutes. Add tofu and continue cooking until heated through, about 5 minutes. Pour in the eggs and jalapeno and cook for 2 minutes. Stir in fresh cilantro just before serving. Serve with fresh avocado and tomatillo salsa if desired.

22 Kale, Mushroom, Onion Breakfast Casserole

Makes 4 servings.

Organic Ingredients:

- 12 oz brown mushrooms (or white mushrooms, but I think the brown ones have more flavor)
- 1 yellow onion
- 2 teaspoons + 2 Tbsps. olive oil
- 8 oz finely chopped kale
- fresh ground black pepper and sea salt to taste
- 10 eggs, beaten until yolks and whites are well-combined

Simple Preparation:
Preheat oven to 375°F. Rub a little olive oil on an 8 1/2 inch x 12 inch glass a baking dish so that the eggs won't stick. Wash and dry mushrooms and thickly slice. Heat 2 Tbsps. olive oil in a large non-stick non-toxic frying pan over medium-high heat, add the mushrooms, and sauté until the mushrooms have released their liquid and it has evaporated, and mushrooms are starting to slightly brown, about 5-6 minutes. Spread out the sautéed mushrooms over the bottom of the baking dish. While the mushrooms cook, chop kale, cutting away the thick stems and chopping the leaves. Add 2 Tbsps. more olive oil to the same pan, heat to medium high, add the chopped kale all at once and sauté, turning kale over and over until it's wilted, about 2-3 minutes. Layer the wilted kale over the mushrooms in the baking dish. Season the vegetables with fresh ground black pepper and sea salt. Beat the eggs until they're well-combined; then pour eggs over the vegetables. Use a fork to gently "stir" until all the ingredients are coated with egg and the top of the casserole shows a good mixture of mushrooms and kale. Bake at 375°F for 40-45 minutes, or until the casserole is completely set and the top is starting to lightly brown. Serve hot. This will keep in the fridge for at least a week.

23 Orange Chia Seed Breakfast Pudding

Makes 2 servings.

Organic Ingredients:

- 1/4 cup almonds, soaked overnight, drained and rinsed
- 1 cup water
- 3 dates, softened with pits removed
- 3 oranges
- 1/3 cup chia seeds

Simple Preparation:
Place almonds and water in high-speed blender. Process until well blended. Remove to nut milk bag and strain. Place almond milk back in blender with dates. Blend until very smooth. Remove the zest from one orange and add to the almond milk date mixture. Segment the insides of the orange and set aside. Juice the two remaining oranges. Add the juice (approximately 1/2 to 3/4 cup) to the almond milk and zest. Stir. Add chia seeds, stir. Let set for 20 minutes. Stir in orange sections that you set aside and enjoy!

24 Sprouted Raw Flaked Oats

Makes about 3 1/2 cups flaked oats.

Organic Ingredients:

- 2 cups organic raw oat groats
- filtered water

Simple Preparation:
Place oats in sprouting jar and fill with water. Soak overnight or for 12 hours. Drain water and rinse 2 more times in the next 12 hours. 24 hours in total. Dry oats in dehydrator at 115 degrees or if it is a warm dry day, outside in the sun on screens. Grind through grain flaker.

25 Morning Muesli

Makes 1 serving.

Organic Ingredients:

- 1/2 cup flaked sprouted oats
- 1 Tbsp. chia seeds
- 1/2 teaspoon cinnamon
- 1/2 cup nut milk (see below)
- 1/2 cup sliced strawberries
- 1/2 cup blueberries
- chopped pecans

Simple Preparation:
Mix oats, chia seeds, cinnamon and nut milk together. Let sit for 1/2 hour. Add fruit and optional nuts and maple syrup. Stir and enjoy!

26 Vegetable Quinoa Bites

Makes 24 bites.

Organic Ingredients:

- 2 cups cooked quinoa
- 2 large eggs
- 3 carrots, shredded
- 1 and 1/2 cups fresh spinach, chopped
- 1 medium shallot, chopped
- 2 teaspoons garlic
- 2 Tbsps. brown rice flour
- Sea salt and pepper, to taste

Simple Preparation:
Preheat the oven to 350°F degrees. Lightly grease your mini muffin pan with olive oil so the bits don't stick. In a large bowl, combine all of the ingredients together, mixing until thoroughly combined. Using a melon baller or a tablespoon, place rounded drops of the mixture into each cup of the muffin pan, pressing each one down lightly with your fingers to make sure that each one is firmly packed. Bake until lightly golden, about 15-20 minutes. Serve immediately.

27 Honey Apricot Millet with Blueberry Compote and Toasted Almonds

Makes 2 servings.

Organic Ingredients:

- 1/2 cup dry millet
- 1/4 cup dried apricots, chopped
- 1/4 cup slivered almonds, toasted
- 2 Tbsps. honey, divided + additional for serving
- 1 cup blueberries + additional for serving
- 1/2 teaspoon fresh lemon juice
- 1/2 teaspoon fresh lemon zest

Simple Preparation:
Rinse millet in a small strainer until water runs clear. In a medium saucepan, toast millet until grains become fragrant, about 3 minutes. When grains are toasted, add 1 cup water to the pot and bring to a boil. When boiling, stir millet once, cover and reduce heat to a simmer. Simmer, covered for 15 minutes. While simmering, combine blueberries, 1 Tbsp. honey, lemon zest, juice, and 3 Tbsps. water in a small saucepan over medium-high heat. Once mixture begins to boil, reduce heat and cook on low for about 10 minutes. While cooking, gently smash blueberries against side of saucepan with a wooden spoon. Allow for mixture to reduce to desired consistency. After millet has simmered for 15 minutes, remove from heat, stir in apricots and 1 Tbsp. honey, let stand, covered for an additional 10 minutes. To serve, spoon millet into a large bowl. Top with sugar free compote, fresh blueberries and toasted almonds.

28 Acorn Squash Quinoa Breakfast Porridge

Makes 4 servings.

Organic Ingredients:

- 1 acorn squash (you will use 1 cup diced)
- 1/2 cup dry quinoa
- 1/2 cup filtered water
- 1/2 cup light unsweetened coconut milk
- pinch of sea salt
- 1/4 cup roasted sunflower seeds
- 1/4 cup chopped walnuts
- 1 Tbsp. olive oil
- 2 Tbsps. virgin coconut oil
- 1 Tbsp. agave syrup (sweeten to taste)
- 1/4 cup dried figs, diced
- 1/4 cup raisins
- 1 cup diced apple

Simple Preparation:

Preheat oven to 425°F with the rack in the middle. Pierce the acorn squash several times with a sharp knife. Bake it for about 45 minutes or until soft and cooked through. Let it cool a bit. Cut it in half, scoop out seeds. Dice flesh into small pieces. Combine the quinoa with water and coconut milk. Bring to a boil, cover and simmer until all of the liquid is absorbed (about 10 to 20 minutes). Stir in the rest of the ingredients and serve hot.

29 Quinoa Apple Breakfast Bites

Makes 2 servings.

Organic Ingredients:

- 2 cups cooked quinoa
- 1 apple, chopped into small pieces
- 3 eggs
- 1/4 cup agave syrup
- 1/2 teaspoon cinnamon
- pinch of salt

Simple Preparation:
Preheat oven to 350°F degrees. Spray a mini muffin pan with cooking spray. Put all ingredients into a medium mixing bowl. Stir until well combined. Scoop mixture into prepared pan. Bake for about 12-13 minutes, just until set. Do not over bake!

30 Ginger Quinoa Granola

Makes 2 servings.

Organic Ingredients:

- 1/2 cup whole almonds
- 1/2 cup walnut pieces
- 1/4 cup flax seeds
- 1/4 cup agave syrup
- 2 Tbsps. coconut oil
- 1 teaspoon cinnamon
- 1/2 teaspoon salt
- 1/3 cup dried ginger pieces, chopped
- 1/3 cup dried cranberries, chopped

Simple Preparation:
Preheat the oven to 350°F. In a large bowl combine the quinoa, almonds, walnuts, and flax seeds and stir well. Heat the agave syrup in a small microwave-safe bowl on high for 20 seconds. Stir in the coconut oil, cinnamon, and salt; continue to stir until the coconut oil is completely melted. Pour the wet ingredients over the dry and toss to coat. Spread the quinoa granola mixture in a thin layer over a parchment line baking sheet. Bake for 20 minutes or until golden brown, stirring twice during the cook time. Add the chopped ginger pieces and cranberries during the last 5 minutes of cook time. Cool completely on the baking sheet, as it cools the granola will harden and begin to clump together. When cooled break up any large pieces of granola into small clusters and store for up to 2 weeks in the refrigerator. Add to a bowl of almond milk and enjoy.

31 Almond Milk Froth

Quick & Easy Milk Froth

Makes 1 serving.

Organic Ingredient:

- Almond Milk

Simple Preparation:
Pour milk into a Mason jar, filling no more than halfway. Secure the lid and shake for 30 seconds. Remove the lid and microwave for another 30 seconds. Using a spoon to hold back the foam, pour the milk into your cup of tea. Scoop the foam on top.

32 Cashew Almond Nut Milk

Makes 1 serving.

Organic Ingredients:

- 1 cup almonds
- 1/2 cup cashews
- 5 cups water

Simple Preparation:
Put all ingredients in blender and blend very well, Strain through nut-milk bag or cheese cloth. You can reserve the nut milk pulp and make flour out of it.

33 Protein-Rich Cranberry-Oat Smoothie

Makes 1 serving.

Organic Ingredients:

- 1/3 cup fresh or frozen unsweetened cranberries
- 1 cup unsweetened rice, almond or soy milk
- small handful raw almonds
- 1 Tbsp. brown rice powder
- 1/2 large fresh pear, cored
- 2 Tbsps. old-fashioned rolled oats (not instant or quick-cook)
- 1 teaspoon cinnamon
- 1-2 lettuce leaves, optional
- 3-5 drops plain or vanilla stevia liquid

Simple Preparation:

Place all ingredients in a high-powered blender and blend until smooth. Drink immediately.

34 Avocado and Melon Smoothie

Makes 1 serving.

Organic Ingredients:

- 2 ripe, fresh avocados
- 1 cup honeydew melon chunks
- 1 ½ tsp. lime juice
- 1 cups almond milk
- 1/2 cup apple juice
- 1 Tbsp. honey

Simple Preparation:
Add all the ingredients to a blender and blend well. Serve cold. Holds well in the refrigerator up to 24 hours. If made ahead, stir gently before pouring into glasses.

35 Avocado Cherry Smoothie

Makes 1 serving.

Organic Ingredients:

- 1 avocado
- 1 green apple, diced
- 1 cup spinach
- 1 banana
- 1/4 cup fresh cherries
- 2 Tbsps. chia seeds
- 1/2 cup filtered water

Simple Preparation:
Add all the ingredients to a blender and blend well. Serve cold. Stores well in the refrigerator up to 24 hours.

36 Berry Chia Smoothie

Makes 2 servings.

Organic Ingredients:

- 1 1/2 to 2 cups almond milk
- 1 banana
- 2 cups frozen blueberries or raspberries
- 1 cup spinach leaves
- 4 teaspoons chia seeds

Simple Preparation:
Simply combine all the ingredients in a blender and blend until smooth.

37 Raspberry-Orange Sunrise

Makes 2 servings.

Organic Ingredients:

- 4 cups fresh orange juice (about 8 oranges)
- 1 cup frozen unsweetened raspberries
- 1 1/2 cups sparkling water
- 3 orange slices, halved

Simple Preparation:
Place orange juice and raspberries in a blender; process until smooth. Pour juice mixture into a pitcher; stir in sparkling water. Serve over ice. Garnish with orange slices.

38 Happy Digestion Smoothie

Makes 2 servings.

Organic Ingredients:

- 1 heaping cup frozen or fresh pineapple chunks
- 1/2 frozen banana
- 1/2 cup water
- 1/2 cup coconut water
- 1/4 cup packed fresh parsley
- 2 Tbsps. avocado
- 1 teaspoon packed freshly grated ginger
- 1/4 teaspoon probiotic powder, optional
- lemon slice, for garnish

Simple Preparation:
Add all ingredients into a blender and blend on the highest speed until super smooth.

39 Apple Pie Smoothie

Makes 2 servings.

Organic Ingredients:

- 1 medium apple, cored and cut in chunks
- 1/2 of one medium cucumber, peeled and cut in chunks
- large handful of spinach, kale, lettuce, or other mild leafy green
- 1/2 medium avocado
- 2 Tbsps. raw pumpkin seeds or walnuts
- 1-2 teaspoons cinnamon, to your taste
- 1/2 teaspoon ground ginger
- 10-15 drops stevia liquid or 1-2 Tbsps. agave nectar
- 1 cup plain or vanilla soy, almond or rice milk, very cold

Simple Preparation:
Place all ingredients in a high powered blender and blend until perfectly smooth (you can use a regular blender, but will likely have to blend in batches, or else use a bit more liquid). The smoothie will be very thick, but if you like it thinner, add more milk or water until desired consistency is reached. Drink immediately.

40 Chocolate Hazelnut Breakfast Smoothie

Makes 2 servings.

Organic Ingredients:

- 1/2 pear, frozen
- 2/3 cup rice milk, plain or chocolate
- 2/3 cup water
- 3 Tbsps. whole hazelnuts, lightly toasted
- 1-1/2 Tbsps. chia seeds
- 1 Tbsp. raw cacao powder (or use cocoa, but increase the stevia)
- 10-15 drops plain or chocolate stevia liquid, to your taste

Simple Preparation:

Place all ingredients in a high-powered blender and blend until smooth. Serve immediately.

CHAPTER 2
Snacks

It's one of the biggest falsehoods in the diet world that snacking leads to weight gain. Eating the wrong kinds of toxic foods in too large quantities can lead to weight gain, but snacking itself is not bad. In fact, teaching children and yourself to snack in a healthy manner can be the best way to lose weight and keep it off. The key, of course, is *healthy* snacking. Eating a bag of potato chips or a spoonful of ice cream is not healthy snacking. That is how extra toxic calories sneak into your diet and make it impossible to lose weight.

However, learning the benefits of healthy snacking and what exactly constitutes a healthy snack can make it much easier to feel full and eat healthy foods throughout the day. Many people grab those unhealthy snacks because they are hungry and therefore susceptible to temptation. When you're hungry the more primitive part of your brain activates which makes it very difficult to think straight and make good choices. If you eat unhealthy snacks, you get pulled into a never-ending spiral of hunger. Because those snacks do not benefit your body, and you will be hungry again in an hour or so, which leads to more snacking, probably, again on unhealthy food.

If you can train yourself to fill hunger with a healthy, filling snack, instead of junk food, you will find reduced calorie and healthy-foods much, *much* more appetizing. The benefits of this type of snacking are multifaceted. First, you prevent yourself from reaching for that bag of chips. If, instead, you eat a handful of almonds or a cup of fresh fruit pieces, you will feel just as full, but you won't be loaded down with toxic chemicals that exhaust the body.

Another benefit of healthy snacking during the day is that you are unlikely to overeat during a meal. Some people allow themselves to overeat at meal time because they abstain from snacking between meals. This "reward" mentality can cause a person to develop a very unhealthy relationship with food. If, instead, you think of food as fuel (and you want to put the very best fuel in your body, to keep it running well), and fuel your body with good fuel when it is hungry, you will be less likely to "save" room for meal times and then "reward" yourself by overeating.

How do you know how often you should eat and what you should eat? Whether it is a meal or a snack, you should eat when you're hungry about every three to four hours. Stick to raw, healthy foods.

Snacks are one of those things that may not currently be planning or thinking about during the day. Do you often find yourself grabbing for something without thinking, without realizing the chemicals you are putting in your body?

You have to remember that when it comes to snacks. They aren't actual meals and you shouldn't treat them as one. Their purpose, essentially, is just to keep your metabolism going. If metabolism shuts down because your body thinks it is starving, you will have an extremely difficult time losing weight.

More and more, companies are stocking vending machines with a few alternative choices such as fruit or nuts. However, if you think that you might get a snack craving while at work or on a trip, it's best to bring along your own choices to avoid any unwanted temptation.

The obvious choice in this category is, of course, nuts. You can carry them in your purse in a bag or small container to have them readily available. You don't have to worry about a mess because they are natural finger foods. Also a bag or container of blueberries make a super snack. Any fruit can fill on the spot, be it an apple or banana. There are healthy suga free bars that will last in your purse or backpack for days.

1 Kale Chips

Makes 4 servings.

Organic Ingredients:

- 1 large bunch of kale, stems removed and leaves chopped into large pieces
- 2 Tbsps. olive oil
- sea salt to taste

Simple Preparation:
Preheat the oven to 350°F. The kale leaves must be SUPER DRY. Toss the dry leaves with olive oil and use your hands to distribute the oil evenly. Then, line a baking sheet with parchment paper and lay some of the leaves on top in a single layer. Make sure the leaves are all flat and not folded over or they won't crisp properly. Bake the kale for 12 minutes. Salt the kale right when you take it out of the oven.

2 Oats and Lentil Vegan Pancakes

Makes 4 servings.

Organic Ingredients:

- 1/2 cup oats
- 1/2 cup red lentils
- 1/4 + 1/2 cup filtered water
- 1 Tbsp. fresh ginger, chopped
- 2 cloves garlic, chopped
- 1/2 teaspoon salt
- 1/2 teaspoon turmeric
- 1/2 teaspoon red chili powder
- 1/2 teaspoon Garam Masala
- 1/4 cup carrots, shredded
- 1/4 cup white onion, chopped finely
- 2 Tbsps. olive oil

Simple Preparation:
Wash the red lentils well with water and then soak them for 15-30 minutes. Grind oats in a coffee grinder to make a fine powder and set it aside. After soaking time is over, grind together lentils, ginger, garlic and 1/4 cup of water into a smooth paste. Transfer it into a bowl. Add powdered oats, salt, turmeric powder, red chili powder & garam masala powder, mix well. Add 1/2 cup of water to make a thin batter for pancake, add carrots and onions, mix well. Heat a non-toxic non-stick pan on medium heat & grease it lightly with olive oil. Spread 1/4 cup batter on the non-stick pan to make a pancake. Cook one side over a slow flame until the base is golden brown in color. Turn over to cook the other side. Remove the pancake and repeat with the remaining batter to make more pancakes. Serve hot with any nutritious chutney, pickle, or enjoy as it is.

3 Baked Butternut Squash Chips

Makes 2 servings.

Organic Ingredients:

- 1 small butternut squash, peeled and halved lengthwise with the seeds removed.
- 2 sprigs of fresh rosemary, finely chopped
- Kosher salt
- Fresh ground black pepper
- Extra virgin olive oil

Simple Preparation:

Preheat your oven to 375°F degrees and begin lining 2 baking dishes with parchment paper. Fill a large pot with water and bring it to a steady, rolling boil. Slice the squash very thinly with a sharp knife. Try to go for 1/2 inch or thinner if at all possible. Boil the squash for approximately 2 minutes. This will have to be done in batches, so don't overcrowd your pot. Lay the squash after boiling onto paper towels. Pat the squash completely dry. This is an essential step and you can't overlook it. The squash needs to be completely dry before moving on. Carefully transfer the dried squash to prepared pans. Make sure it's a single layer. Don't overlap the squash in any way. Brush the tops of the squash with extra virgin olive oil and sprinkle with sea salt and black pepper. Season them to taste and then add rosemary to the top. Bake for approximately 20 minutes, checking at the halfway mark to make sure you aren't burning them. If your slices are on the thinner side, they won't need the entire time to cook so checking is important! Remove them when they are starting to brown and crisp up. Apply more salt to taste and serve immediately.

4 Spicy Roasted Chickpeas

Makes 2 cups.

Organic Ingredients:

- 2 cups cooked chickpeas
- 1/4 teaspoon of sea salt
- 1 1/2 teaspoon extra virgin olive oil
- 1/4 teaspoon black pepper
- 3/4 teaspoon turmeric
- 1/4 teaspoon paprika
- 1/4 teaspoon garlic powder
- A bit of cayenne to taste

Simple Preparation:

Preheat your oven to 425°F. Mix your seasonings (salt, pepper, turmeric, paprika, garlic powder, and cayenne) in a small bowl, making sure they are well combined. Cover baking sheets with parchment paper. How many you need will be determined by the size of the baking sheet. Pat the chickpeas dry and make sure and remove any loose skins. Brush the chickpeas with the olive oil and sprinkle your seasoning mixture over the top. You might need to roll them around or toss them to coat them completely. Bake them for 25 minutes, stirring them near the halfway mark.

5 Apricot and Seed Protein Bars

Makes 6 servings.

Organic Ingredients:

- 2/3 cup dried apricots
- 1/3 cup oats
- 1/3 cup desiccated coconut
- 1/4 cup sunflower seeds
- 1 Tbsp. sesame seeds
- 1/4 cup dried cranberries
- 3 Tbsps. hemp protein powder
- 1 Tbsp. chia seeds

Simple Preparation:
Purée apricots in a food processor with 2/3 cup boiling water and the oats, then scrape the mixture into a bowl. Toast coconut, sunflower seeds and sesame seeds in a non-stick pan over a low heat, then stir into the apricots with the cranberries, hemp powder and chia seeds to make a thick paste. Roll into a long log on a sheet of cling film. Wrap tightly, chill, and then slice thinly to serve. Will keep in the fridge for 2 weeks.

6 Simple Hummus

Makes 2 cups.

Organic Ingredients:

- 4 garlic cloves
- 2 cups canned chickpeas, drained, liquid reserved
- 1 1/2 teaspoons kosher salt
- 1/3 cup tahini (sesame paste)
- 6 Tbsps. freshly squeezed lemon juice (2 lemons)
- 2 Tbsps. water or liquid from the chickpeas
- 8 dashes hot sauce

Simple Preparation:
Turn on the food processor fitted with the steel blade and drop the garlic down the feed tube; process until it's minced. Add the rest of the ingredients to the food processor and process until the hummus is coarsely pureed. Taste, for seasoning, and serve chilled or at room temperature. Drizzle with olive oil.

7 Lemon and Coriander Hummus

Makes 4 servings.

Organic Ingredients:

- 2, 15 oz cans chickpeas in water, rinsed and drained
- 3 garlic cloves, roughly chopped
- 3 Tbsps. tahini paste
- 3 Tbsps. extra-virgin olive oil, plus extra for drizzling on top
- zest and juice 2 lemons
- 2 Tbsps. ground coriander
- sea salt

Simple Preparation:
Put everything but the coriander into a food processor, then whizz to a fairly smooth mix. Scrape down the sides of the processor if you need to. Season the hummus generously, then add the coriander and pulse until roughly chopped. Spoon into a serving bowl, drizzle with olive oil, then serve.

8 Faux Biscuits

Makes about one dozen 3-inch biscuits.

Organic Ingredients:

- 3/4 cup dairy-free milk (I use almond milk or coconut milk; dairy milk will work fine, too, for a non-vegan version)
- 1/2 cup hummus
- 1 cup almond flour, packed
- 2/3 cup tapioca flour
- 2 teaspoon baking powder
- 1/4 teaspoon salt
- 2 teaspoon coconut flour

Simple Preparation:

Preheat oven to 450°F. Grease or line one large baking sheet with parchment paper. In a large bowl, add milk and then hummus, stirring until fairly well mixed. Add almond flour, tapioca flour, baking powder, and salt. Mix well. Add coconut flour. Mix and let sit for about 3 to 5 minutes, until batter is visibly thicker---like biscuit dough---when stirred. Drop a heaping teaspoon of batter onto the baking sheet and then drop a little more on top of that. That second dollop of batter on top the first is important. Without it, your biscuits will be too thin and cook too quickly. When dropped, batter will not spread past a 3-inch radius, and will not spread further when baked. So batter for the biscuits may be dropped fairly close together. Bake for about 10 to 12 minutes. Tops will take on a light golden appearance and look done, and bottoms of biscuits will be a nice even brown.

9 Smashed Celeriac

Makes 2 servings.

Organic Ingredients:

- 1 celeriac, peeled
- 3 Tbsps. olive oil
- 1 handful fresh thyme, leaves picked
- 2 cloves garlic, finely chopped
- sea salt
- freshly ground black pepper
- 3-4 Tbsps. water or organic vegetable stock

Simple Preparation:
Slice about 1/2 inch off the bottom of the celeriac. Dice it into 1/2 inch cubes. Put a casserole-type pot on a high heat, add 3 Tbsps. of olive oil, then add the celeriac, thyme and garlic, with a little seasoning. Stir around to coat and cook quite fast, giving a little color, for 5 minutes. Turn the heat down to a simmer, add the water or stock, place a lid on top and cook for around 25 minutes, until tender. Season carefully to taste and stir around with a spoon to smash up the celeriac.

10 Seeded Oatcakes

Makes 8 servings.

Organic Ingredients:

- 5 oz medium oatmeal
- 5 oz oats
- 4 oz plain flour
- 1/2 teaspoon black pepper
- 1/2 teaspoon sea salt
- 2 oz seeds (mix of sunflower, poppy seeds & sesame)
- 3 oz olive oil

Simple Preparation:
Preheat the oven to 350°F. In a large bowl mix together the oatmeal, porridge oats, black pepper, salt and seeds. Pour over the olive oil and mix until combined. Add 5 oz of warm water adding a little more if necessary to bring it to a firm dough. Dust a surface and two baking sheets with flour. Roll out the dough to ¼ in then cut out 24 rounds with a 2¾ in cookie cutter. Roll the edges of the oatcakes through a shallow saucer of water. Then roll through poppy seeds to coat the edges. Place on the prepared baking sheets and transfer to the oven for 20 minutes. Cool on a wire rack. Store in an airtight container.

11 Roasted Brussel Sprouts with Garlic Aioli

Makes 2 servings.

Organic Ingredients:

- Garlic Aioli sauce (see below)
- 1 pound fresh brussel sprouts
- 3 Tbsps. olive oil
- sea salt and pepper

Simple Preparation:
Preheat oven to 400°F. Cut off the brown ends of the Brussels sprouts and pull off any yellow outer leaves. Cut them into quarters. Mix them in a bowl with the olive oil, salt and pepper. Pour them on a sheet pan and roast for 35 to 40 minutes, until crisp on the outside and tender on the inside. Shake the pan from time to time to brown the sprouts evenly. Serve immediately with garlic aioli.

12 Garlic Aioli

Makes 2 servings.

Organic Ingredients:

- 4 garlic cloves
- 2 large egg yolks
- 5 teaspoons fresh lemon juice
- 1 teaspoon Dijon mustard
- 1/2 cup extra-virgin olive oil

Simple Preparation:
Mince and mash garlic to a paste with a pinch of salt using a large heavy knife. Whisk together yolk, lemon juice, and mustard in a bowl. Add olive oil, a few drops at a time, to yolk mixture, whisking constantly, until all oil is incorporated and mixture is emulsified. Whisk in garlic paste and season with salt and pepper. If aioli is too thick, whisk in 1 or 2 drops of water. Chill, covered, until ready to use.

13 Hearty Granola Bars

Makes 12 servings.

Organic Ingredients:

- 1 1/2 cups mashed ripe banana
- 1 teaspoon pure vanilla extract
- 2 cups rolled oats
- 3/4 cup dried cherries, chopped
- 1/2 cup almonds, chopped
- 1/2 cup sunflower seeds
- 1/2 cup pepita seeds
- 1/2 cup sliced almonds
- 1/4 cup hulled hemp seeds
- 1 teaspoon cinnamon
- 1/4 teaspoon sea salt to taste

Simple Preparation:
Preheat the oven to 350°F. Lightly grease a large rectangular baking dish (8 in by 12 in) and line with a piece of parchment paper so the bars are easier to lift out. In a large bowl, mash the banana until smooth. Stir in the vanilla. Place the rolled oats into a food processor and pulse until the oats are coarsely chopped but still have with lots of texture. Stir oats into the banana mixture. Chop the almonds and cherries and stir these and the rest of the ingredients into the banana-oat mixture until thoroughly combined. Spoon mixture into prepared dish. Press down until compacted and smooth out with hands until even. Use a pastry roller to smooth out if desired. Bake for 25 minutes until firm and lightly golden along the edge. Place dish on a cooling rack for 10 minutes then carefully slide a knife to loosen the ends and lift out. Place granola slab on a cooling rack for 10 minutes and then into the freezer for another 10 mins. Slice into bars once they are cool.

14 Chana Masala Spiced Roasted Nuts

Makes 6 servings.

Organic Ingredients:

- 3 cups mix of cashews, pecans, walnuts, almonds, pistachios
- 2 teaspoons olive oil
- 1 teaspoon chole masala (see below)
- 1/2 teaspoon salt and black pepper to taste

Simple Preparation:
In a large wide pan, add the olive oil and heat on low-medium. When hot, add the nuts, salt, black pepper and chole masala spice to taste, and mix to coat well. Roast the nuts stirring every few seconds for about 10 minutes until the cashews start to look golden. Be careful not to burn the nuts. Take them off the heat. The omega-3 fats in the nuts can burn and damage easily, so roast them to just a light golden. Cool completely, adjust salt and spice. You can also bake these for about 12 minutes in the oven at 330°F degrees.

15 Chole Masala Spice

Makes 1 serving.

Organic Ingredients:

- 2 Tbsps. cumin seeds
- 1 teaspoon turmeric powder
- 1 Tbsp. coriander seeds
- 1/2 Tbsp. black peppercorns
- 10 cloves
- 1 Tbsp. sesame seeds
- 10 green cardamom pods
- 4 black cardamom pods
- 1/2 Tbsp. ginger powder
- 1 Tbsp. amchur powder
- 5 cinnamon sticks
- 2 bay leaves
- 1 star anise
- 1/2 teaspoon nutmeg
- 1/2 Tbsp. sea salt
- Simple Preparation:

Dry roast all the ingredients. Allow it to cool, then grind and store it in an airtight container.

16 Scallion Pancakes

Makes 4 servings.

Organic Ingredients:

- 8 oz cauliflower
- 1/4 cup water
- 1/4 cup scallions, chopped
- 1/4 cup onion, chopped finely
- 2 eggs
- 1/4 teaspoon sea salt
- 2 Tbsps. coconut oil

Simple Preparation:

Begin by preparing your cauliflower. Manually cut into coarse florets then mince through a food processor. If you don't have a food processor, you may also mince your cauliflower through a vegetable grater. In a large saucepan fitted with a lid, heat up 1/4 cup of water until it is boiling. Immediately place all of the minced cauliflower in the saucepan, give it a quick stir, cover and turn off the heat. Let steam for exactly 10 minutes. Once the 10 minutes is up, remove the cauliflower from the saucepan into a fine mesh bag and squeeze all of the moisture out. Move the strained cauliflower into a small bowl and set aside. Crack two eggs into a small bowl. Whisk the eggs with a fork, then toss it, along with the scallions, onion, cauliflower and 1/4 teaspoon of sea salt in a medium bowl until well combined. In a large frying pan, heat up 2 Tbsps. of oil on medium heat, then place all of the egg mixture into the pan. Spread it out with a spatula to evenly cover the whole pan. Let cook for about 5 minutes or until golden brown. Flip the pancake by sliding the pancake (browned side still down) from the pan onto a large plate, invert the pan onto the plate and flip both together back onto the stove, making it so that the uncooked side is now at the bottom. Cook for another 3 minutes or so, until also golden brown. Slide the pancake from the pan to a large plate and cut into 6 pieces. Sprinkle with more sea salt and serve hot.

17 Avocado Baked Eggs

Makes 2 servings.

Organic Ingredients:

- 2 ripe avocados
- 4 fresh eggs
- 1/8 teaspoon pepper
- 1 Tbsp. chopped chives

Simple Preparation:
Preheat the oven to 425°F degrees. Slice the avocados in half, and take out the pit. Scoop out about two tablespoons of flesh from the center of the avocado, just enough so the egg will fit in the center. Place the avocados in a small baking dish. Do your best to make sure they fit tightly. Crack an egg into each avocado half. Try your best to crack the yolk in first, then let the egg whites spill in to fill up the rest of the shell. Place in the oven and bake for 15 to 20 minutes. Cooking time will depend on the size of your eggs and avocados. Just make sure the egg whites have enough time to set. Remove from oven, then season with pepper, chives, and garnish of your choice.

18 Spirulina Hemp Bars

Makes 6 servings.

Organic Ingredients:

- 1/2 cup pistachios
- 1/2 cup pumpkin seeds
- 3/4 cup shredded coconut
- 1/4 cup orange juice
- 1/4 cup hemp hearts
- 1/4 cup coconut oil
- 1/2 tsp spirulina powder
- 3/4 cup dates, chopped

Simple Preparation:
In a food processor, pulse the ingredients until the mixture is crumbly but beginning to come together. Press into an 8-inch square cake pan or glass dish. Chill in the refrigerator for at least an hour, then slice and serve.

19 Maple Roasted Parsnips

Makes 6 servings.

Organic Ingredients:

- 1 pound parsnips
- 1/4 cup coconut oil, melted
- 3 Tbsps. real maple syrup

Simple Preparation:
Preheat the oven to 400°F. Peel the parsnips and cut them into chip sized pieces and place into an oven proof roasting dish. Pour over the coconut oil and distribute evenly. Drizzle over the maple syrup and stir to combine well. Place in the oven and cook for 15 minutes. Remove from the oven and toss the parsnips over to allow the other side to brown. Place back in the oven and cook for a further 10 to 15 minutes or until golden.

20 Fruit Leather

Makes 6 servings.

Organic Ingredients:

- 2 apples, finely diced
- 10 strawberries, diced
- 1 ruby pink grapefruit, diced
- Stevia/rice malt syrup to sweeten if needed
- 1 teaspoon cinnamon
- Pinch sea salt
- 1/4 cup water

Simple Preparation:

Place the fruit in saucepan with the water and bring to a boil. Reduce the heat and simmer until the fruit is soft and the liquid has been reduced. Stir through the cinnamon and salt. Transfer the fruit to a blender and puree until smooth. Taste the mixture and if required add a sweetener. The grapefruit can be quite tart and while suitable for adults, children may not appreciate this. If you would like a sweeter roll up than I suggest adding some sweetness to balance out the sourness. If a sweetener is added blend again until combined. You should end up with 2-3 cups worth of pureed fruit. Line a large baking tray with parchment paper. Pour the mixture onto the tray and spread it out thinly by using the back of a spatula. You want it to just cover the baking paper's surface without leaving any gaps (the thinner the better!). Place the baking tray in the oven on the lowest shelf available and bake for 8-12 hours. Leave to bake overnight at about 250F for 9 hours. Remove the tray from the oven and using a sharp knife cut the fruit leather into strips. Let it cool completely before peeling the fruit leather off the baking paper. Roll up if desired and store in an airtight container for up to a week.

21 Rosemary Almonds

Makes 6 servings.

Organic Ingredients:

- 2 cups raw almonds
- 2 Tbsps. fresh rosemary, minced
- 2 teaspoons salt (or to taste, depending on how salty you like nuts)
- 4 Tbsps. olive oil

Simple Preparation:
Place the almonds in boiling water for 1 minute to blanch (not any longer than that). Remove the almonds from the boiling water and run them under cold water to cool. Shake the water off in a colander, and then pop the skins off with your fingers. Heat a large pan over medium heat. Add enough olive oil to generously coat the bottom of your pan (approx. 3-4 tablespoons), and allow to heat up. Add the almonds to the pan. Stir frequently so that the almonds don't burn. The almonds will be ready when they're golden brown (approx. 5-7 minutes). Turn down the heat to low and add the rosemary and salt. Stir well, and cook just until the rosemary becomes fragrant (approx. 2 minutes). Remove the almonds from the pan and place on paper towel to drain any remaining oil.

22 Sweet Potato Balls

Makes 6 servings.

Organic Ingredients:

- 1 medium size cooked sweet potato
- 2 cups almond meal
- 1 teaspoon vanilla
- 3 teaspoons baking powder
- 3 egg yolks
- 4 Tbsps. melted coconut oil
- 1-2 teaspoons honey
- 3 Tbsps. coconut flour
- 1 cup of unsweetened shredded coconut and coconut flakes

Simple Preparation:
Peel and mash the cooked sweet potato until smooth. Mix in the almond meal, vanilla and baking powder until everything is incorporated. Mix in the wet ingredients including the egg yolks, melted coconut oil and honey. Stir the mixture until everything is combined. Add 3 Tbsps. coconut flour. Notice the mixture will be less wet but not too dry. Do not try to put too much coconut flour as it absorbs a lot of moisture and the balls would be too dry and flaky. Line a baking sheet with a parchment paper. Pre-heat the oven to 350°F. Shape the balls into a ping-pong ball size and roll each of them in the bowl of unsweetened shredded coconut and coconut flakes. The dough will be a little bit sticky but not too sticky that you can't even shape the balls. If it's too sticky, you can add a little more coconut flour. Bake the balls in the oven for about 25 minutes or until the edges turn golden brown or they are dried out already. Remove them from heat and let them cool down. The balls are soft when they're still warm but as they cool down, they should become more firm. After they've cooled down, store the balls in the refrigerator.

CHAPTER 3
Lunch and Dinner

Lunch is the midpoint of your day so you might not need too much to keep you going, especially if you have healthy snacks available throughout the day. However, you can't simply forego the meal completely. Your body needs nutrition and vitamins just as badly at noon as it does at 8 AM or 6 PM. However, you should make sensible choices.

A salad is filling and healthy, and using a balsamic vinegar/extra virgin olive oil dressing is best. You can always mix it up, by adding things like slivered almonds or roasted chickpeas. You can even add berries.

Using whole grain wraps, you can put various legumes and vegetables into an easy to carry pouch. Don't skimp on the vegetables, especially the greens.

There is also soup. Which are healthy, hearty, and are especially easy to heat up or even eat cold. The following are just a few of my favorite recipes.

When it comes to dinner, people tend to fall into two camps - they either want comfort food or something light. Fortunately for many people, unlike with lunch, you have the luxury of being able to cook at home. You might be exhausted and want nothing more than to pop something in the microwave and sit in front of the television. However, you must fight that temptation. And remember, just because it's home cooking, doesn't mean it must take long.

What time of day do you eat dinner? If your life is like most working American's, you might not get home from work until six, which means, if you want to cook yourself a meal, you might not eat until seven or eight, depending on what you want to cook. Eating this late in the day, especially if you are trying to go to bed early to get up for another full day of work, can be very bad for your system.

Per a recent study published by the *International Journal of Obesity*, participants who ate their largest meal early in the day (and most people eat their largest meal at dinnertime), lost far more weight than those who waited until later in the day to eat even if they were eating about the same number of calories. Both were on diets designed to help them lose weight.

The participants in the study were required to keep their sleeping and physical activity habits about the same, so that the only real variation was when they were eating. Over the course of the study, those that ate early dinners before 6PM lost more than twenty pounds. The study showed that people who ate later were more likely to also skip breakfast in the morning, which leads to overeating later in the day. Also, early eaters not only lost more weight, but their meal cycle and sleep cycle were better aligned, so they slept better, had less heartburn, and lower levels of bad cholesterol, better hand-eye coordination, and had better glucose levels. Eating your larger meal earlier in the day can mean a much more natural life rhythm that improves sleep and lowers stress.

I've found that I lose the most weight when I eat dinner at 6 pm and then don't eat anything else that night.

1 Delicious Garbanzo Bean Salad

Makes 4 serving.

Organic Ingredients:

- 15 oz can garbanzo beans (Make sure the can says BPA Free lining or use dried beans.)
- 2 ripe avocados
- 1 lemon
- 1 small red onion
- 1 small red pepper
- 1/4 cup extra virgin olive oil (Californian is best.)
- 1 handful of fresh basil
- 1 Tbsp. dried cumin
- 1 Tbsp. dried turmeric

Simple Preparation:
Place a strainer in the sink. Open the can of garbanzo beans and pour them into the strainer. Rinse the beans well until you no longer see bubbles. If you do not rinse the beans, all the gas will go into your stomach, which is very unpleasant. Place the beans in clean water in a pot on the stove and bring to a boil. Then drain them in the strainer again. Rinse the ripe avocados and place them on a cutting board. Cut open the avocados and remove the skin and the large seed in the middle. Dice the avocados into pieces the size of a small marble - approximately 1/4 inch square. Some people like a lot of red onion and some people don't. I recommend starting with less, because you can always add more to suit your personal taste. Dice the red onion into tiny pieces. Chop the red pepper into small pieces of a similar size to the avocado. Chop the fresh basil into small ribbons. Squeeze out the juice of one lemon into a large bowl. Add to the bowl your garbanzo beans, avocados, red onion, red pepper, basil, cumin, turmeric, and olive oil. Enjoy!

2 Quinoa Fruit Medley

Makes 6 servings.

Organic Ingredients:

- 3 cups quinoa
- 4 cups vegetable broth
- 2 cups filtered water
- 1 cup olive oil
- 1/2 cup fresh lemon juice
- the zest of 1 lemon
- 1 cup dried apricots, chopped into small pieces
- 1 cup dried cherries
- 1 cup dried cranberries
- 1 green apple diced
- 1/2 cup cilantro minced
- 1 teaspoon curry powder
- sea salt and black pepper

Simple Preparation:
In a large pot bring the vegetable broth and water to a boil. Add your quinoa and cook for 15 minutes. After the first 10 minutes have passed, add the apricots, cherries and cranberries to the boil so that they soften up a little. Once the quinoa has finished cooking, take it off the heat and let cool. Stir in the olive oil, lemon juice, lemon zest, cilantro, green apple, curry powder, and some salt and pepper. Enjoy!

3 Chimichurri Rice and Lentils

Makes 6 servings.

Organic Ingredients:

- Chimichurri Sauce (see below)
- 1 cup lentils
- 1 cup brown rice
- 1 cup wild rice
- 4 cups vegetable broth
- 2 cups filtered water
- 3 bay leaves
- sea salt and black pepper

Simple Preparation:
In a large pot bring the vegetable broth and water to a boil. Add the brown rice and wild rice and bay leaves. Cook for 45 minutes. After 35 minutes have passed, add the lentils. Once the rice and lentils have finished cooking, remove the bay leaves and season with sea salt and pepper to taste. Place each serving in a bowl and mix in one or two tablespoons of Chimichurri Sauce to your individual taste preference.

4 Chimichurri Sauce

Makes 4 servings.

Organic Ingredients:

- 1 bunch flat leaf parsley
- 8 cloves garlic, minced
- 3/4 cup extra virgin olive oil
- 1/3 cup lemon juice
- 1 tablespoon diced red onion
- 1 teaspoon dried oregano (optional)
- 1 teaspoon black pepper
- 1/2 teaspoon salt

Simple Preparation:
Place parsley, garlic, lemon juice, red onion, oregano, salt, and pepper (to taste) in the bowl of a food processor fitted with a blade attachment. Process until finely chopped, stopping and scraping down the sides of the bowl with a rubber spatula as needed, about 1 minute total. With the motor running, add oil in a steady stream. Scrape down the sides of the bowl and pulse a few times to combine. Transfer sauce to an airtight container and refrigerate at least 2 hours or up to 1 day to allow the flavors to meld. Before serving, stir and season as needed. The chimichurri will keep in the refrigerator for up to 1 week.

5 Lemony Spinach Garbanzo Bean Salad

Makes 8 servings.

Organic Ingredients:

- 2, 15 oz cans garbanzo beans (Make sure the can says BPA Free lining or use dried beans.)
- 1 oz bag of baby spinach
- 1 green apple diced into small pieces
- 1 lemon - juiced
- 1/2 cup dried cherries
- 1/4 cup preserved lemon rind minced (see recipe below)
- 1/4 cup extra virgin olive oil (Californian is best.)
- 1 teaspoon dried cumin
- pinch of sea salt to taste

Simple Preparation:
Place a strainer in the sink. Open the cans of garbanzo beans and pour them into the strainer. Rinse the beans well until you no longer see bubbles. If you do not rinse the beans, all the gas will go into your stomach, which is very unpleasant. Place the beans in clean water in a pot on the stove and bring to a boil. Then drain them in the strainer again. Pour the beans back into the pot or in a large bowl for mixing. Add the diced green apple, the minced preserved lemon rind, the olive oil, the cumin, lemon juice and cherries. Pour over fresh baby spinach and enjoy!

6 Preserved Lemon Rind

Fills a 1 quart jar.

Organic Ingredients:

- 6 - 8 whole lemons
- 4 Tbsps. sea salt

Simple Preparation:
Start by cleaning your quart jar in hot soapy water. Dry with a clean towel. Clean the outsides of the lemons, rinse and pat dry. Slice the ends from the lemons to create a flat top and bottom. Stand the lemon on one of the flat ends. To preserve the lemons whole, cut an "x" in the lemon and stop when you are about 1/2 inch from cutting all the way through. The quarters of the lemon remain attached at the base. Open the lemon and pour in 1/2 Tbsp. of salt. Don't worry if some of the salt spills out. Once you salt the lemons, pack them into the jar as tightly as possible. You can use a pestle or a wooden spoon to push them in. Once all of the lemons are in the jar, add an additional 1 Tbsp. of salt. Press on the lemons one more time to extract as much juice as possible. If the lemons are submerged in juice you can secure the lid, if not you may need to add additional fresh lemon juice to top them off. Use a pestle to press on the lemons and extract as much juice as possible. Top off the jar with fresh lemon juice if needed. Seal the jar and store the lemons in a cool dry place for at least 1 week. Give them a shake every once in a while to disperse the juice and salt. After 1 week, move your lemons to refrigerator. When the peels become translucent, you will know they are soft and ready for use. When you are ready to use a lemon, remove it from the jar and rinse to remove excess salt. Cut all of the remaining lemon flesh and pith away from the rind and discard. You can store the lemons in the refrigerator for up to 6 months. Both Meyer and regular lemons work well and provide slightly different flavors. Have fun and experiment by adding a cinnamon stick, a bay leaf, a couple of peppercorns and a couple of coriander seeds to each jar.

7 Kale and Quinoa Salad with Dates, Almonds and Citrus Dressing

Makes 6 servings.

Organic Ingredients:
For the salad and toppings:

- 1 Tbsp. olive oil
- 1 large onion, diced
- sea salt to taste
- 1/2 cup red quinoa
- 1 small clove garlic, smashed
- 1 pound lacinato kale, tough stems removed
- ¾ cup whole dates
- 1/2 cup roasted salted whole almonds

For the dressing:

- 1 clementine or mandarin orange, juiced
- 1/2 lime, juiced
- 2 teaspoons honey
- 1/4 cup extra-virgin olive oil
- Salt and freshly ground black pepper

Simple Preparation:
Heat the olive oil in a wide sauté pan over medium heat. Add the onion and sprinkle lightly with salt. Cook, stirring occasionally, until the onion has darkened to a toasty brown and smells caramelized — about 20 minutes. Remove from the heat and set aside. You should have about 1/2 cup of cooked onions. Rinse the quinoa in a fine mesh strainer. Add it and the garlic to a 2-quart saucepan set over medium-high heat and sauté for about a minute both to dry the grain and toast it lightly. Add 1 cup water and 1/2 teaspoon salt and bring to a boil. Cover and turn the heat to low; cook for 15 minutes. Turn off the heat but leave the lid on for an additional 5 minutes. After 5 minutes, remove the lid and fluff with a fork. While the onions are caramelizing and the quinoa is cooking, then slice the kale into fine ribbons. Wash thoroughly and spread on a towel to dry. Pit the dates and slice them into quarters. Roughly chop the almonds.

To make the dressing:
Whisk the juices together. Whisk in the honey and olive oil. The dressing will be emulsified but still thin. Stir the dressing into the quinoa after it finishes cooking. Toss the kale with all of the still-warm quinoa and the caramelized onions. Toss with about half the dressing and taste. Add the remaining dressing if desired, then toss with the dates and almonds. Refrigerate for up to 5 days.

8 Crunchy Winter Salad

Makes 4 servings.

Organic Ingredients:

- 2 cups carrots, chopped
- 1 small celeriac, peeled and chopped
- 1 red onion, sliced
- 1/3 cup chopped mixed nuts, walnuts, hazelnuts or pecans are good
- 4 Tbsps. olive oil
- 2 Tbsps. red wine vinegar
- 1 teaspoon Dijon mustard

Simple Preparation:
Peel the carrots and celeriac and grate in a food processor. Mix together with the onion and nuts. Whisk the oil and vinegar with some mustard, salt and pepper and toss with the salad immediately to stop the celeriac going brown. Cover and keep in the fridge for up to a day.

9 Roasted Butternut Squash Salad with Warm Cider Vinaigrette

Makes 4 servings.

Organic Ingredients:

- 1 1/2-pound butternut squash, peeled, seeds removed and 3/4-inch diced
- ¼ cup olive oil
- 1 Tbsp. agave syrup
- sea salt and freshly ground black pepper
- 3 Tbsps. dried cranberries
- 3/4 cup apple cider or apple juice
- 2 Tbsps. apple cider vinegar
- 2 Tbsps. minced shallots
- 2 teaspoons Dijon mustard
- 4 oz baby arugula, washed and spun dry
- 1/2 cup walnuts halves, toasted

Simple Preparation:

Preheat the oven to 400°F. Place the butternut squash on a sheet pan. Add 2 tablespoons olive oil, the agave syrup, 1 teaspoon salt and 1/2 teaspoon pepper and toss. Roast the squash for 15 to 20 minutes, turning once, until tender. Add the cranberries to the pan for the last 5 minutes. While the squash is roasting, combine the apple cider, vinegar, and shallots in a small saucepan and bring to a boil over medium-high heat. Cook for 6 to 8 minutes, until the cider is reduced to about 1/4 cup. Off the heat, whisk in the mustard, 1/2 cup olive oil, 1 teaspoon salt, and 1/2 teaspoon of pepper. Place the arugula in a large salad bowl and add the roasted squash mixture, the walnuts, and the grated Parmesan. Spoon just enough vinaigrette over the salad to moisten and toss well. Sprinkle with salt and pepper and serve immediately.

10 Vegetable Tagine with Almond and Chickpea Couscous

Makes 4 servings.

Organic Ingredients:

- 1 1/2 cups shallots, peeled and cut in half
- 2 Tbsps. olive oil
- 1 large butternut squash, about 2 lb 12 oz, peeled, deseeded and cut into bite size chunks
- 1 teaspoon ground cinnamon
- ½ teaspoon dried ginger powder
- 2 cups vegetable stock
- 12 small pitted prunes
- 2 teaspoons honey
- 3 Tbsps. chopped coriander
- 2 Tbsps. chopped mint, plus extra for sprinkling

For the couscous:

- 1 cup dried couscous
- 1 Tbsp. cumin
- 1 Tbsp. chili powder
- 15 oz can chickpeas, rinsed and drained
- handful toasted flaked almonds

Simple Preparation:
Cook the shallots in the olive oil for 5 mins until they are softening and browned. Add the squash and spices, and stir for 1 min. Pour in the vegetable stock, season well, then add the prunes and honey. Cover and simmer for 8 mins. Stir in the coriander and mint. Pour 1 1/2 cups boiling water over the couscous in a bowl, then stir in the cumin and chili powder with 1/2 teaspoon of salt. Pour in the chickpeas, then cover and leave for 5 mins. Fluff up with a fork and serve with the tagine, flaked almonds and extra mint.

11 Barley, Kale and Vegetable Soup

Makes 4 servings.

Organic Ingredients:

- 1 onion, chopped
- 2 garlic cloves, crushed
- 1 cup barley
- 1/4 cup water
- 2 cups carrots, peeled and diced
- 1 parsnip, peeled and diced
- 1 turnip, peeled and diced
- 1 tablespoon dry thyme or a handful fresh
- 1/2 teaspoon coriander seeds
- 8 cups vegetable stock
- 1 bay leaf
- A large handful of flat leaf parsley, chopped
- 1 small bunch kale

Simple Preparation:

Place chopped onion and garlic in a large 4 quart soup pot. Add 1/4 cup water and bring to a boil. Cook stirring until the water almost evaporates. Add the carrots, parsnip, and turnip and stir them around for a couple of minutes. Add the thyme and coriander seeds. Add the rinsed barley and the vegetable stock and bring to a boil. Lower the heat, and add half the parsley and cook, partially covered, until barley is cooked and the vegetables are tender. When the soup is done add the ribboned kale and cook another three minutes or so. Adjust seasoning and serve or store in mason jars to serve later.

12 Crunchy Cucumber and Radish Salad

Makes 1 serving.

Organic Ingredients:

- 1/2 cucumber
- 1/2 bunch radishes
- 2 Tbsps. olive oil
- 1 teaspoon lemon juice

Simple Preparation:
Thinly slice the cucumber and radishes, and arrange on a plate. Whisk together the olive oil and lemon juice, and drizzle over the vegetables to serve.

13 Herbed Spaghetti Squash

Makes 4 servings.

Organic Ingredients:

- 1 small spaghetti squash, about 2 1/4 pounds
- 2 1/2 Tbsps. olive oil
- 2 1/2 Tbsps. finely chopped mixed soft herbs, such as basil, chives, chervil, parsley and sage
- 1/2 teaspoon sea salt
- 1/8 teaspoon freshly ground black pepper

Simple Preparation:
Preheat the oven to 375°F. Using a sharp knife, cut the squash in half lengthwise and place, cut side down, in a baking dish. Add enough water to come 1/2 inch up the sides of the baking dish and cover with aluminum foil. Bake for 45 minutes, until the squash is easily pierced with a paring knife. Turn squash over and cover with foil again and continue to cook another 15 minutes, until the squash is very tender. Remove from the oven, uncover, and allow to cool slightly. Using a spoon, remove the seeds and discard. Using a fork, gently pull the strands of squash away from the peel and place the squash strands into a mixing bowl. Heat a skillet. Add the olive oil, spaghetti squash, herbs, salt and pepper and toss thoroughly but gently to heat and combine. Serve immediately or cover and keep warm until ready to serve.

14 Squash and Coconut Curry

Makes 4 servings.

Organic Ingredients:

- 2 Tbsps. Madras curry paste (see below)
- 1 large butternut squash (1 lb 5oz peeled weight), chopped into medium size chunks
- 1 red onion
- 13 1/2 oz can coconut milk
- small bunch coriander, roughly chopped

Simple Preparation:
Heat a large frying pan or wok, add the curry paste and cook for 1 min. Add the squash and onion, and then toss well in the paste. Pour in the coconut milk with 2/3 cup water and bring to a simmer. Cook for 15 - 20 mins or until the butternut squash is very tender and the sauce has thickened. Season to taste, then serve.

15 Madras Curry Paste

Makes ½ cup.

Organic Ingredients:

- 2 1/2 Tbsps. coriander seeds, dry-roasted and ground
- 1 Tbsp. cumin seed, dry roasted and ground
- 1 teaspoon brown mustard seeds
- 1/2 teaspoon cracked black peppercorns
- 1 teaspoon chili powder (such as cayenne - not the SW seasoning)
- 1 teaspoon ground turmeric
- 2 crushed garlic cloves
- 2 teaspoons grated fresh ginger
- 3 - 4 tablespoons lemon juice

Simple Preparation:
Put all ingredients except the lemon juice into small bowl and mix together well. Add the lemon juice and mix to a smooth paste. Keep for up to one month in an airtight container in fridge.

16 Kale Salad with Apricots and Avocado

Makes 1 serving.

Organic Ingredients:

- 8 oz kale
- 8 dried apricots, chopped
- 1/3 cup cooked white beans
- 1/4 cup almonds
- 1 Tbsp. olive oil
- 2 Tbsps. lemon juice
- 1/2 avocado
- salt and pepper

Simple Preparation:
Fold a piece of kale in half lengthwise and use your fingers to tear out the tough inner stem. Repeat with the other leaves of kale (you can save the stems to use in stir-fries, sauces, or soups). Tear all the leaves into bite-sized pieces and put them in a medium-sized mixing bowl. Add the apricots to the bowl with the kale, along with the beans, and the almonds. Whisk together the oil and vinegar (or shake it in a small canning jar). Pour the vinaigrette and a pinch of salt over the salad and use your fingers to toss and rub everything together. Transfer the salad to a bowl or a lunch container (if eating later). Just before eating, slice the avocado into cubes and spoon them over the salad. This salad will keep for about 24 hours, preferably refrigerated.

17 Cauliflower Curry Soup

Makes 6 servings.

Organic Ingredients:

- 2 Tbsps. olive oil, plus more to serve
- 2 medium white onions, thinly sliced
- 1/2 teaspoon sea salt
- 1 large head of cauliflower (about 2 pounds), trimmed and cut into florets
- 4 1/2 cups low-sodium vegetable broth (or water)
- 1/2 teaspoon coriander
- 1/2 teaspoon turmeric
- 1 1/4 teaspoon cumin
- 1 cup coconut milk
- Freshly-ground black pepper, to season
- 1/4 cup roasted cashew halves, for garnish
- 1/4 cup finely chopped Italian parsley, for garnish

Simple Preparation:

Heat oil in a large pot over medium heat until shimmering. Cook the onions and 1/4 teaspoon salt until onions are soft and translucent, or about 8-9 minutes. Reduce heat to low, add garlic and cook for 2 additional minutes. Add cauliflower, vegetable broth, coriander, turmeric, cumin, and remaining 1/4 teaspoon salt. Bring pot to a boil over medium-high heat, then reduce the heat to low. Simmer until cauliflower is fork-tender, about 15-17 minutes. Working in batches, purée the soup in a blender until smooth, and then return the soup to the soup pot. (Alternatively, use an immersion blender to purée the soup right in the pot.) Stir in the coconut milk and warm the soup. Taste and add more salt, pepper or spices if you'd like. To serve, ladle the soup into favorite bowls and garnish with a handful of toasted cashews, a few sprigs of parsley, and a dash of olive oil to top.

18 Spring Rolls

Makes 6 servings.

Organic Ingredients:

- 1/4 cup dried Asian mushrooms, soaked to rehydrate
- 1/4 cup thin brown rice noodles, cooked
- 1 cup Chinese cabbage, finely sliced
- 1 carrot, peeled and julienned
- 3 spring onions, white parts sliced on the diagonal, green parts finely sliced into ribbons
- 1 inch piece of ginger, peeled and grated
- 1 large bunch of Thai basil, roughly chopped
- 1 large bunch of coriander, roughly chopped
- 1/2 cup fresh beansprouts
- 16 large brown rice spring roll wrappers, thawed if frozen
- 10 mint leaves
- Hoisin sauce

Simple Preparation:
Lay one spring roll wrapper into a shallow dish of warm water and carefully place onto cutting board. Place 1/4 cup rice noodles in center of wrapper. Top with mushroom, cabbage, carrot, spring onion, Thai basil, ginger, coriander, and 1-2 mint leaves. Roll lengthwise from the bottom, fold in each end, and then roll over tightly. Slice in half. Proceed with the rest of the spring roll wrappers. Keep refrigerated until ready to serve. Serve with hoisin sauce.

19 Spring Rolls

Makes 6 servings.

Organic Ingredients:

- 1/2 cup vermicelli brown rice noodles
- 1/3 cup kale
- 1/4 cup beansprouts
- 1 carrot
- 1 tablespoon pickled ginger
- 1 large pomegranate
- 4 sprigs of fresh mint
- 4 sprigs of fresh coriander
- 1 Tbsp. olive oil
- 12 medium round brown rice-paper wrappers

For the Honey Sweetened Dipping Sauce:

- 4 Tbsps. Wheat free Tamari soy sauce
- 1 spring onion
- 2 Tbsps. almond butter
- 1 Tbsp. honey
- 2 Tbsps. brown rice vinegar
- 1/4 teaspoon garlic powder
- 2 teaspoons olive oil

Simple Preparation:
To make the dipping sauce, trim and finely chop the spring onion. Place into a small bowl with the remaining sauce ingredients and 1 Tbsp. of water, then mix well. Taste and adjust the flavors, if needed. Prepare the noodles according to the packet instructions. Drain, then leave to cool. Cut away any tough stalky bits from the kale, finely slice and place into a large bowl with the cooled noodles and beansprouts. Peel and slice the carrot into thin batons, roughly a half inch in length, then add to the bowl. Finely slice and add the ginger. Cut the pomegranate in half, hold one half over the bowl, cut-side down, and bash the back of it with a wooden spoon so that all of the

seeds come tumbling out. Repeat with the other half. Pick in the herb leaves and add the olive oil, then toss well. Dip one of the rice paper wrappers in a shallow bowl of warm water. Allow to soak for around 10 seconds until soft and pliable, drain on kitchen paper, then place onto a board. Spoon 1 heaped tablespoon of the filling onto the wrapper in a rough line, about a half inch from the edge nearest to you (be careful not to overfill them as they'll be hard to roll). Fold the edge nearest to you over the filling, then tightly roll it away from you, tucking in the left and right edges as you go, then press down to seal. Repeat with the remaining ingredients, halve each roll at an angle, then serve with the dipping sauce.

20 Carrot Pittas

Makes 6 servings.

- Organic Ingredients:
- 6 medium carrots
- a bunch of fresh coriander
- 2 Tbsps. sesame seeds
- 1 Tbsp. poppy seeds
- 6 brown rice pitas
- 1 orange
- 2 lemons
- extra virgin olive oil
- sea salt
- freshly ground black pepper
- tahini dressing (see below)

Simple Preparation:
Preheat the oven to 250°F. Peel the carrots on a chopping board. Pick the coriander leaves and finely chop them, discarding the stalks. Place a small non-stick frying pan on a medium heat, add the seeds and leave them to toast for 3 to 4 minutes, or until lightly golden, tossing regularly, then tip them into a salad bowl. Coarsely grate the carrots using a box grater, then add them to the salad bowl along with the coriander leaves. Pop the pittas onto a baking tray and into the oven for a few minutes to warm through. To make the dressing, use a microplane to finely grate the zest of the orange, then add it to a small mixing bowl. Cut the orange in half and squeeze in the juice, catching any seeds with your hand. Cut the lemons in half and squeeze in the juice from 1½ lemons, then add 5 Tbsps. of extra virgin olive oil. Add a tiny pinch of salt and pepper, then mix well with a fork. Pour the dressing into the salad bowl and toss everything together well, adding a squeeze more lemon juice if you think it needs it. Use oven gloves to remove the pittas from the oven, then serve with the zingy salad and some homemade tahini dressing and let everyone stuff and build their own pittas.

21 Tahini Dressing

Makes 2 servings.

Organic Ingredients:

- 1 cup sesame seeds
- 2 tablespoons or more olive oil
- Salt (optional)

Simple Preparation:
Toast raw sesame seeds. On the stovetop, place the sesame seeds in a dry skillet over medium heat, stirring them frequently with a wooden spoon. Toast the seeds until they are lightly colored (not brown) and fragrant, about 5 minutes. Transfer the toasted sesame seeds to a large plate or tray and let them cool completely. Place the sesame seeds in a food processor fitted with the S-blade. Grind the sesame seeds: Process for 2 to 3 minutes until the sesame seeds form a crumbly paste. Add 2 tablespoons of olive oil to the food processor. Process for 1 to 2 minutes, scraping down the sides as necessary, until the mixture forms a thick and fairly smooth paste. For thinner tahini, add more oil, 1 to 2 tablespoons at a time, and process until the desired consistency is reached. Add salt to taste and process until combined. Store the tahini: Transfer the tahini to a jar or other airtight container. Store it in the refrigerator for a month or longer. If the mixture separates, stir the tahini to redistribute the oil.

22 Green Bean Curry

Makes 4 servings.

Organic Ingredients:

- 2 cups brown basmati rice
- 3 cups filtered water
- 16 oz extra firm sprouted tofu, cut into 1 inch square cubes
- 4 Tbsps. olive oil
- 1 yellow onion, chopped
- 2 cups fresh or frozen green beans
- 13 1/2 oz can of coconut milk
- 1 Tbsp. Thai green curry paste
- 2 Tbsps. fresh ginger minced
- 2 Tbsps. fresh garlic minced
- 0.8 oz can sliced bamboo shoots
- 3 Tbsps. liquid aminos or soy sauce
- sea salt to taste

Simple Preparation:
Cook the rice according to the directions on the package. If there aren't any directions, then put brown rice and water together in a pot with a lid. Use the ratio of 1 1/2 cups water to 1 cup rice. Set the heat to maximum, and bring the rice/water to a boil uncovered. Turn off the heat, and let the rice sit in the covered pot for another 10 minutes. In a large skillet heat the olive oil over medium high heat and brown the tofu on all sides. When the tofu is ready remove it from the skillet and place it on a paper towel so that the extra oil is absorbed. Add your onions to the hot skillet and when they are starting to turn translucent and the garlic and ginger. Cook for a minute or two. Don't let the garlic burn. Then add the bamboo shoots, coconut milk, green beans, Thai green curry paste and liquid aminos or soy sauce. Simmer for 8 minutes to thicken the sauce and then add your cooked tofu. Serve over the cooked brown basmati rice.

23 Creamy Barley and Squash Risotto

Makes 6 servings.

Organic Ingredients:

- 1 Tbsp. olive oil
- 1 onion, finely chopped
- 1 small butternut squash, peeled and diced into small chunks
- 2 garlic cloves, crushed
- 1 2/3 cups pearl barley
- 6 cups hot vegetable stock
- large handful parsley, chopped

Simple Preparation:
Heat the olive in a large shallow saucepan. Add the onion and squash, and cook very gently, stirring occasionally, until the onion is soft and the squash is starting to soften, about 10 mins. Stir in the garlic and cook for 1 min more. Add the barley, give it a stir and pour in the stock. Gently simmer for 45 mins, stirring occasionally, until all the stock has been absorbed and the barley is tender. Add a little extra stock during cooking if it evaporates too quickly. Turn off the heat and stir in all the parsley, then season.

24 Microwave Butternut Squash Risotto

Makes 2 servings.

Organic Ingredients:

- 1 cup brown risotto rice
- 3 cups hot vegetable stock
- 1 medium butternut squash
- handful sage leaves, roughly chopped

Simple Preparation:
Tip the rice into a large bowl, then add 2 cups of the hot vegetable stock. Cover with cling film and microwave on High for 5 mins. Meanwhile, peel and cut the squash into medium chunks. Stir the rice, then add the squash and the rest of the stock. Re-cover with cling film, then microwave for another 15 mins, stirring halfway, until almost all the stock is absorbed and the rice and squash are tender. Leave the risotto to sit for 2 minutes. Every microwave is different, so adjust cooking time accordingly.

25 Brown Rice Mushroom Risotto

Makes 4 servings.

Organic Ingredients:

- 3 Tbsps. olive oil, divided
- 1 small yellow onion, chopped
- 2 cloves garlic, pressed or minced
- 5 cups vegetable broth, divided
- 1 1/2 cups brown Arborio/short-grain brown rice
- 14 oz sliced baby Portobello mushrooms
- 2 Tbsps. olive oil
- 2 teaspoons tamari
- 1 teaspoon sea salt, more to taste
- Freshly ground black pepper, to taste
- 4 sprigs fresh oregano, leaves removed from stems and larger leaves torn into small pieces

Simple Preparation:
Make sure your oven rack is in the middle position. Preheat oven to 375°F degrees. Heat 1 Tbsp. olive oil in a medium Dutch oven over medium heat until shimmering. Add onion and a pinch of salt. Cook, stirring occasionally, for ten minutes, then add the minced garlic. Cook for another 2 to 4 minutes, until the onions are well browned. Add 4 cups broth, cover, and bring to a boil over medium-high heat. Remove from heat and stir in the rice. Cover the pot and bake until rice is tender and cooked through, about 60 to 65 minutes. During the last 20 minutes of baking time, prepare the mushrooms. Warm 2 Tbsps. olive oil in a large skillet until shimmering. Add the cleaned, sliced mushrooms to the pot with a dash of salt. Cook, stirring occasionally, until the mushrooms are darker in color, fragrant and have soaked up most of their own juices, about 13 minutes. Remove the pot from the oven. Pour in the remaining cup of broth, olive oil, tamari, salt, and a generous amount of pepper. Stir vigorously for 2 to 3 minutes, until the rice is thick and creamy. Stir in the mushroom mixture and any remaining juices. Season to taste with salt and pepper, divide into bowls and top with a generous sprinkling of torn, fresh oregano leaves.

26 Roasted Cauliflower and Brussel Sprouts

Makes 4 servings.

Organic Ingredients:

- 1 1/2 lb Brussels sprouts, cut in half
- 4 cups cauliflower, cut into bite size pieces
- 10 cloves peeled garlic
- 2 Tbsps. olive oil
- 1/8 teaspoon salt
- 1/8 teaspoon black pepper

Simple Preparation:
Preheat oven to 400°F degrees. Coat the brussels sprouts, garlic and cauliflower with olive oil, salt and pepper. Spread the vegetables on a large baking pan. Bake vegetables for 30 minutes, stirring occasionally, until the vegetables are tender. Serve over brown rice.

27 Arugula and Chickpea Salad with Lemon Dill Vinaigrette

Makes 4 servings.

Organic Ingredients:

- 1/3 cup olive oil
- 3 Tbsps. freshly squeezed lemon juice
- 1 Tbsp. minced fresh dill
- 1 small garlic clove, finely chopped
- Coarse sea salt or kosher salt and freshly ground black pepper
- 3 bunches arugula, trimmed and roughly chopped
- 1 can white beans, such as cannellini or Great Northern, rinsed and drained
- 1 yellow bell pepper, halved, seeded and thinly sliced

Simple Preparation:
In a large bowl, whisk together the oil, lemon juice, dill, garlic, and salt and pepper. Add the arugula, beans, and yellow pepper and toss to combine.

28 Warm Pear Spinach Salad

Makes 2 servings.

Organic Ingredients:

- 1 Tbsp. extra virgin olive oil
- 1 medium white onion, thinly sliced
- 1/2 bunch spinach, washed and roughly chopped
- salt and pepper to taste
- 1-2 pears washed, cored and thinly sliced
- 1/4 cup sunflower seeds

Simple Preparation:
In a skillet heat the olive oil until it just begins to shimmer. Add onions and cook over a low heat stirring often until onions take on a deep golden color and begin to caramelize, which could take 20 minutes or so. Remove from pan and set aside. Once you have washed the spinach, just leave the water on it and add it to the skillet. Cook until just wilted which only takes a couple of minutes. Add salt and pepper to taste and a bit more olive oil if it seems too dry. Plate the spinach and top with sliced pears, onions and sunflower seeds. Serve warm or at room temperature.

29 Couscous Salad with Cucumber Red Onion and Herbs

Makes 4-6 servings.

Organic Ingredients:

- 1 cup couscous
- 1 1/4 cups boiling water
- 1 cup loosely packed cilantro, finely chopped
- 1 cup loosely packed Italian parsley, finely chopped
- 1/2 cucumber, cut lengthwise and very thinly sliced
- 1/2 red onion, cut in half and shaved extremely thin
- 1 lemon, zested and juiced, about 3 tablespoons
- 1/4 cup extra-virgin olive oil
- 1 Tbsp. honey or agave syrup, warmed
- 1/2 teaspoon chili powder
- 1/2 teaspoon ground cumin
- 3 tablespoon toasted pine nuts
- Salt and pepper to taste

Simple Preparation:
Put the couscous in a large bowl and pour the boiling water over it. Cover with a lid and set aside for 5 minutes. Then remove the lid and fluff with a fork. Toss the finely chopped herbs with the couscous, as well as the sliced cucumber, onion, and lemon zest. Whisk together the lemon juice, olive oil, honey, chili powder, and cumin, then toss this dressing with the couscous. Stir in the pine nuts. Taste and season with salt and pepper. Serve immediately, or refrigerate until ready to serve. Store leftovers in a covered container for up to 5 days.

30 Curried Tofu Salad

Makes 4-6 servings.

Organic Ingredients:

- 1/3 cup golden raisins
- 1 teaspoon yellow mustard seeds
- 1/4 cup apple cider vinegar
- 1 pound extra firm tofu
- 2 Tbsps. roasted pumpkin seeds
- 1 scallion, chopped
- 1 tablespoon chopped parsley
- 1/2 cup vegan mayonnaise (see below)
- 2 Tbsps. curry powder
- 3/4 teaspoon kosher salt
- Freshly ground black pepper

Simple Preparation:
Place the raisins and mustard seeds in a small heatproof bowl. Bring the apple cider vinegar to a boil and pour it over the raisins and mustard seeds. Let them soak for at least 10 minutes or longer. Rinse and drain the tofu and gently press it between towels to rid of excess water. Place the tofu in a large bowl and roughly crumble it using your hands or a fork. Add the raisins and mustard seeds (along with any excess vinegar), pumpkin seeds, scallions, and parsley. In a separate bowl, stir together the mayonnaise, curry powder, salt, and pepper to taste. Add this to the tofu mixture and stir until thoroughly combined. Taste and adjust seasonings if desired. Serve as a sandwich spread or on a bed of salad greens. To store, refrigerate in an airtight container for up to 3 days.

31 Vegan Soy Mayonnaise

Makes 3 cups.

Organic Ingredients:

- 2 1/4 cups olive oil
- 1 cup soymilk
- 1 Tbsp. agave nectar
- 3/4 teaspoon sea salt (to taste)
- 2 - 2 1/2 teaspoons apple cider vinegar, raw or 2 1/2 teaspoons lemon juice, fresh squeezed
- 1/2 teaspoon Dijon mustard

Simple Preparation:
Combine all ingredients except vinegar or lemon juice in blender, blending until smooth. Slowly add vinegar or lemon juice until liquid thickens.

32 Raw Almond Mayonnaise

Makes 1 cup.

Organic Ingredients:

- 1/2 cup soaked almonds (soak almonds for 8 hours and drain)
- 1/2 cup water
- Juice of 1/2 lemon
- 1/4 teaspoon dried mustard powder
- 1/2 teaspoon salt
- 1/4 teaspoon freshly ground pepper
- 3/4 cup olive oil

Simple Preparation:
Place all the ingredients except the olive oil in a blender and blend until very smooth. With blender still on, carefully and slowly pour a thin stream of olive oil through the opening in the blender's cover. Start with 1/2 cup of oil and continue until you reach the right consistency, up to 3/4 cup. Taste and adjust seasonings, adding more lemon juice or some apple cider vinegar if you want more tanginess.

33 Vegan Tofu Mayonnaise

Makes 1 cup.

Organic Ingredients:

- 12 oz firm sprouted tofu
- 5 Tbsps. water
- 5 Tbsps. olive oil
- 2 Tbsps. lemon juice
- 1/2 teaspoon salt

Simple Preparation:
Whirl all ingredients together in a blender, starting with the lesser amounts of oil and water, adding more if needed until smooth. Taste and adjust seasonings.

34 Edamame Quinoa Salad

Makes 4 servings.

Organic Ingredients:

- 1 1/2 cups frozen edamame, cooked according to package directions
- 2 cups red cabbage, shredded
- 2 cups cooked quinoa
- 3/4 cup diced pineapple
- 1/4 cup raisins
- 2 teaspoons almonds, chopped
- 2 Tbsps. apple cider vinegar
- 2 Tbsps. olive oil
- 1 teaspoon agave syrup
- 1 teaspoon chili powder
- 3 cloves garlic, minced

Simple Preparation:
In a large bowl combine edamame, cabbage, quinoa, pineapple, raisins and almonds. In a small bowl combine vinegar, olive oil, agave syrup, chili powder and garlic. Toss with quinoa mixture and serve either chilled or at room temperature.

35 Kale Salad with Spicy Tempeh

Makes 4 servings.

Organic Ingredients:

- 8 oz tempeh
- 1/4 cup olive oil
- 1/4 teaspoon salt
- 2 teaspoons onion powder
- 2 teaspoons garlic powder
- 1 teaspoon chili powder
- 1 teaspoon lemon pepper
- 1/8 teaspoon cayenne pepper (optional)
- Smoked sea salt (optional)
- 1 lb kale, chopped
- 1 cup shredded carrots
- 15 1/2 oz can chickpeas
- 2 Tbsps. toasted sesame seeds
- 1/3 cup rice vinegar
- 1/4 cup soy sauce or liquid aminos
- 1 Tbsp. fresh grated ginger

Simple Preparation:

Blanch kale in salted boiling water for about 30 seconds. Run it under cold water and drain. Once it cools, squeeze out the excess water and set aside. Preheat oven to 425°F. Combine all salt, onion powder, garlic powder, chili powder, lemon pepper, cayenne pepper in a small bowl and pour in the olive oil. Cut the tempeh into thin slices and then dip each slice in spiced olive oil and arrange them on a baking sheet lined with parchment paper. Bake at 425°F for about 20 minutes, until golden brown and crispy (keep an eye so they don't burn!). Sprinkle with some smoked sea salt. Combine all kale, carrots, and chickpeas in a large bowl. Combine all dressing ingredients (toasted sesame seeds, rice vinegar, soy sauce or liquid aminos, and fresh grated ginger) in a glass jar, close the lid and shake well. Pour over salad and toss until all the ingredients are coated with the dressing. Crumble tempeh on top right before serving.

36 Cumin Lime Black Bean Quinoa Salad

Makes 4 servings.

Organic Ingredients:
For the salad:

- 3 cups cooked quinoa
- 15 oz can black beans, drained and rinsed
- 1 1/2 cups cilantro, finely chopped
- 3 small/medium carrots, julienned
- 4 green onions, chopped
- fine grain sea salt & black pepper, to taste

For the dressing:

- 3 Tbsps. fresh lime juice (about 1 lime)
- 2 Tbsps. olive oil
- 1 large clove garlic, minced
- 1 teaspoon ground cumin
- 1 teaspoon agave syrup
- 1/2 teaspoon fine grain sea salt

Simple Preparation:
In a large bowl, toss the quinoa, black beans, cilantro, carrots, and green onions. Whisk together the dressing in a small bowl or jar. Pour onto salad and toss to combine. Season with salt and pepper to taste.

37 Vegetable Couscous with Chickpeas and Preserved Lemons

Makes 4 servings.

Organic Ingredients:
For the broth:

- 8 1/2 cups vegetable stock
- 2 Tbsps. cumin
- 2 Tbsps. chili powder
- 3 carrots, chopped
- 3 large parsnips, chopped
- 2 red onions, cut into wedges through the root
- 1/2 butternut squash, chopped into chunks
- 4 leeks, sliced into rings
- 12 dried figs, halved

For the couscous:

- 1 cup dried couscous
- 15 oz can of chickpeas
- 4 Tbsps. olive oil
- salt and pepper to taste
- 1 red onion, finely diced
- 3 spring onions, sliced
- 2 Tbsps. cumin
- 1/4 cup olive oil
- 1 lemon, juiced
- bunch coriander, roughly chopped
- 2 preserved lemons, homemade (see recipe) or bought, rinsed, pulp scooped out and finely sliced
- small bunch mint, chopped

Simple Preparation:
For the broth, bring the vegetable stock to a simmer in a large pan. Add the cumin, chili powder and vegetables, bring back to the boil, then reduce heat and simmer for

15 mins. Add the figs and continue to cook for 5 mins more until they are tender. Meanwhile, put the couscous and half the chickpeas into a bowl, add 4 Tbsps. olive oil, and season with salt and pepper. Pour 1 ½ cups boiling water over the couscous, cover and set aside for 10 minutes, then fluff up with a fork. In a separate bowl, combine the red onion, spring onions, cumin, olive oil, remaining chickpeas, lemon juice, preserved lemons, and coriander, then mix into the couscous. Pile onto a large deep serving dish, ladle over the braised vegetables and broth, and sprinkle with the chopped mint.

38 Vegan Chili

Makes 4 servings.

Organic Ingredients:

- 1 1/2 Tbsps. olive oil
- 2 heaping cups diced sweet onion
- 2 Tbsps. minced garlic (about 4 med/lg cloves)
- 2 jalapeños, seeded (if desired) and diced
- 1 cup diced celery
- 1 cup vegetable broth
- 15 oz can kidney beans, drained and rinsed
- 15 oz can pinto beans, drained and rinsed
- 2 Tbsps. chili powder
- 2 teaspoons ground cumin
- 1 teaspoon dried oregano
- 1/2 teaspoon fine grain sea salt to taste
- 1/4 teaspoon ground cayenne pepper

Toppings:

- Chopped green onions
- Fresh cilantro

Simple Preparation:
In a large pot, sauté the onion and the garlic in the oil over medium heat until soft and translucent, about 5 minutes. Season with a pinch of salt and stir. Add the jalapeños and celery and sauté for another 5 minutes, until softened. Add the drained and rinsed beans, along with the chili powder, cumin, oregano, salt, and cayenne. Simmer the mixture until thickened, about 10-15 minutes and adjust seasonings to taste if necessary. Serve with chopped green onion, and cilantro leaves, if desired.

39 Tofu Sweet Potato Soup

Makes 4 servings.

Organic Ingredients:

- 8 cups not-chicken broth
- 14 oz firm tofu, cut into 1 inch cubes
- 3 oz can of green chilies diced
- 1 large bunch of cilantro, chopped
- 1 medium red onion, diced
- 2 medium jalapeño, diced with seeds removed
- 2 cloves of garlic, chopped
- 2 medium sweet potatoes, cut into small bite-sized pieces
- 2 teaspoon thyme
- 3 Tbsps. olive oil
- Salt & Pepper to taste

Garnishes:

- Sliced radishes
- Lime slices
- Cilantro
- Coconut Cream (see below)
- Guacamole (see below)

Simple Preparation:
Heat a tablespoon of olive oil over medium heat. Add tofu and cook until starting to brown on all sides. Season with thyme and set aside. While the tofu browns, cut the garlic, onion & jalapeño. Also, chop the cilantro, peel & chop the sweet potatoes and set both aside. Heat a tablespoon of olive oil over medium heat. Add garlic, onion & jalapeño. Cook until softened. Transfer the garlic, onion & jalapeño into a blender or Cuisinart. Add canned green chilies & chopped cilantro. Blend until smooth. Pour the mix into a stock pot and cook over medium heat, stirring continuously, for 3 minutes until the mix darkens. Add the tofu and not-chicken broth to the stock

pot. Bring to a slow boil or simmer. Add the diced sweet potatoes and cook until fork tender (about 10 minutes). Serve with sliced radishes, additional chopped cilantro, jalapeño, and coconut cream. Or, top with a tablespoon of guacamole.

40 Coconut Cream

Makes 2 servings.

Organic Ingredients:

- 14 oz can coconut cream
- 2 Tbsps. lemon juice
- sea salt to taste

Simple Preparation:
Refrigerate a can of full fat coconut cream overnight (or at least for a few hours). Turnover and open the can to find the heavier fat solids in a layer. Remove the thicken cream, add the lemon juice, and a pinch of salt, mix, and use like sour cream.

41 Guacamole

Makes 2 servings.

Organic Ingredients:

- 3 Haas avocados, halved, seeded and peeled
- 1 lime, juiced
- 1/2 teaspoon kosher salt
- 1/2 teaspoon ground cumin
- 1/2 teaspoon cayenne
- 1/2 medium onion, diced
- 1/2 jalapeno pepper, seeded and minced
- 1 tablespoon chopped cilantro
- 1 clove garlic, minced

Simple Preparation:
In a large bowl place the scooped avocado pulp and lime juice, toss to coat. Drain, and reserve the lime juice, after all of the avocados have been coated. Using a potato masher add the salt, cumin, and cayenne and mash. Then, fold in the onions, jalapeno, cilantro, and garlic. Add 1 tablespoon of the reserved lime juice. Let sit at room temperature for 1 hour and then serve.

42 Lentil Loaf

Makes 4 servings.

Organic Ingredients:

- 1/3 cup red lentils
- 1/2 cup green lentils
- 1 1/2 cups vegetable stock
- 1 bay leaf
- 1 Tbsp. olive oil
- 1 onion, finely chopped
- 1 garlic clove, minced
- 4 1/2 oz mushrooms, finely chopped
- 1 cup carrots, finely chopped
- 1 1/4 cups chopped toasted almonds, divided
- 2 eggs, lightly beaten
- 2 Tbsps. chopped cilantro leaves
- Zest and juice of 1/2 lemon
- Freshly ground pepper

Simple Preparation:

Wash the lentils and put into a large saucepan with the stock and bay leaf. Bring to a boil, then reduce the heat and simmer for 20 to 30 minutes, or until the lentils are soft and all the fluid has absorbed. Preheat oven to 350°F. Line a loaf pan with non-stick parchment paper. Heat the oil in a saucepan or large deep frying pan and sauté the onion and garlic for 2 minutes, or until the onion is soft. Add the mushrooms and carrots and cook for 2 minutes. Remove the bay leaf and add the lentil mixture to the pan, along with the almonds (reserving about 1/4 cup of the almonds), cilantro, lemon zest and juice. Season with salt and pepper and mix well. The mixture should be soft, but not runny. Spoon the lentils into the prepared pan, sprinkle with reserved breadcrumbs over the top, and bake for 35-40 minutes, or until firm to the touch. Remove from the oven and allow to cool in the pan for 10 minutes before turning out. Serve hot or cold

43 Mushroom Bourguignon

Makes 2 servings.

Organic Ingredients:

- 3 Tbsps. extra-virgin olive oil
- 1 small yellow onion, finely chopped
- 3 garlic cloves, crushed
- 1 teaspoon dried thyme
- 2 large Portobello mushrooms, sliced
- 2 1/2 cups button, brown or cremini mushrooms, sliced
- 1/2 cup cooked brown lentils
- 1 cup pomegranate juice
- 1 Tbsp. balsamic vinegar
- 1 tablespoon almond flour
- 2 1/2 cups vegetable stock
- 1 cup pearl onions, peeled
- 1 pinch salt and pepper to taste

Simple Preparation:
In a large, heavy skillet, heat the olive oil. Add the onions and sauté them until they soften, about 3 minutes. Add the garlic, thyme and mushrooms and cook the mixture until the mushrooms soften and begin to brown. Add the lentils and cook for about 2 minutes, then add the pomegranate juice and balsamic vinegar. Continue to cook for 7-10 minutes, or until the liquid has almost cooked off. Sprinkle the flour over the mixture and stir to evenly blend it in. Add in the vegetable stock. Bring the mixture to a simmer and cook, stirring often, for about 10 minutes or until the sauce is thick and dark and the mushrooms are tender. You can adjust the thickness of the sauce by adding in stock to thin it. While the mixture is simmering, drizzle a small skillet with olive oil and place it over medium-high heat. Add in the pearl onions and sauté them until they are soft and begin to brown. Add them into the mushroom mixture, give everything a stir, and taste to adjust salt and pepper seasoning. Serve the bourguignon hot over roasted vegetables, brown rice, cooked barley or quinoa.

44 Avocado and Mango Salsa

Makes 4 servings.

Organic Ingredients:

- 2 cups diced ripe mango (about 2 mangos)
- 1/2 cup finely diced red onion
- 1 cup diced Hass avocado (1 medium avocado)
- 1/4 cup minced fresh cilantro
- 2 tablespoons extra virgin olive oil
- freshly ground black pepper
- big pinch of kosher salt
- 1/4 teaspoon red pepper flakes
- Juice from 1 lime

Simple Preparation:
Combine all the ingredients into a bowl and stir to combine.

45 Roasted Acorn Squash with Quinoa and Mint Salad

Makes 6 servings.

Organic Ingredients:

- 2 acorn squash, halved lengthwise and seeded
- 2 Tbsps. olive oil
- Salt and freshly ground pepper
- 1 cup quinoa
- 2 Tbsps. raisins
- 1 Tbsp. apple cider vinegar
- 1 teaspoon agave nectar
- 1 Granny Smith apple, peeled and finely diced
- 1 large shallot, minced
- 1 garlic clove, minced
- 2 Tbsps. chopped mint
- 2 Tbsps. chopped parsley
- 2 cups arugula

Simple Preparation:
Preheat the oven to 350°F. Season the inside of the squash halves with a little salt and pepper, and place them cut side down on a baking sheet lined with parchment paper. Roast for about 25 minutes, or until tender. As the squash is cooking, bring 2 cups of water to a boil in a medium saucepan. Stir in the quinoa, cover and simmer for 10 minutes. When the quinoa is almost completely done, stir in the raisins and cover for about 5 more minutes or until all the water is absorbed. Pour the quinoa into a large bowl allow it to cool completely, stirring every so often to speed the process along. In a small bowl, whisk the vinegar, agave nectar and olive oil. Pour the dressing over the cooled quinoa and add the green apple, shallot, garlic, mint and parsley. Toss to thoroughly combine. Add the arugula and toss gently once or twice more. After the acorn squash has cooled completely, cut just a little piece off the bottom of each squash half so that it will sit upright on a plate. Set the squash halves on plates and fill the cavity with the salad.

46 Hoisin Sesame Salad with Baked Tofu

Makes 1 serving.

Organic Ingredients:

- 1/3 cup olive oil
- 3 Tbsps. apple cider vinegar
- 2 Tbsps. hoisin sauce (see below)
- 1 Tbsp. toasted sesame seeds
- 1 scallion, minced
- 3 cups mixed greens
- 3/4 cup cubed baked tofu
- 1/2 cup edamame
- 1/2 cup carrot matchsticks or slices
- 1/2 cup sliced snap peas

Simple Preparation:
Place olive oil, vinegar, hoisin sauce, edamame, sesame seeds and scallion in a bowl or a jar with a tight-fitting lid; whisk or shake until well combined. Place greens in an individual salad bowl; toss with 2 tablespoons of the dressing. Refrigerate the remaining dressing. Top the greens with tofu, carrots and snap peas.

47 Hoisin Sauce

Makes 2 servings.

Organic Ingredients:

- 4 Tbsps. liquid aminos
- 2 Tbsps. creamy almond butter
- 1 Tbsp. honey
- 2 Tbsps. apple cider vinegar
- 1 garlic clove, finely minced
- 2 Tbsps. tahini
- 1 teaspoon cayenne
- 1/8 teaspoon black pepper

Simple Preparation:
Combine all ingredients in a small mixing bowl. Mix with a whisk until well blended.

48 Oven Baked Sweet Potato Fries

Makes 6 servings.

Organic Ingredients:

- 2 large garnet yams
- 2 Tbsps. of coconut oil, melted
- sea salt
- freshly ground pepper
- cinnamon

Simple Preparation:

Preheat the oven to 400°F. Peel the yams and cut them into even matchsticks. Then, place them on a foil-lined baking tray (line with parchment paper for a crisper exterior) and toss with the coconut oil, salt, pepper, and cinnamon. Bake for 30 minutes, flipping the frites and tray halfway through. Cook until they are tender in the middle and browned on the edges.

49 Cardamom Carrot Soup

Makes 6 servings.

Organic Ingredients:

- 1 Tbsp. coconut oil
- 2 large leeks, white and light green ends only, cleaned, trimmed, and thinly sliced
- sea salt
- 1 1/2 pounds large carrots, peeled and cut into ½-inch coins
- 1/4 cup diced Braeburn apple
- 1 teaspoon minced fresh ginger
- 1/2 teaspoon ground cardamom
- 4 cups not-chicken broth
- 1/2 cup full-fat coconut milk
- black pepper

Simple Preparation:
Melt the coconut oil in a saucepan over medium heat. Add the leeks, along with a generous pinch of salt, and sauté until translucent, about 5 minutes. Toss in the carrot, apple, ginger, and cardamom, and stir until fragrant. Pour in the broth and bring to a boil over high heat. Turn down the heat to low. Cover and simmer until the carrots are easily pierced with a fork, about 30 minutes. Mix in the coconut milk. Transfer the soup in batches to a blender and process until smooth. Alternatively, purée the soup directly in the pot with an immersion blender. Season with salt and pepper to taste.

50 Sweet Potato Hash

Makes 2 servings.

Organic Ingredients:

- 1 large sweet potato
- 1 teaspoon sea salt
- black pepper
- 1 teaspoon garlic, minced
- 1 Tbsp. onion, minced
- 1 Tbsp. Herbes de Provence
- 2 Tbsps. olive oil

Simple Preparation:
Peel and cut the sweet potato lengthwise so the slices fit in the feeding tube of your food processor. Attach the julienne slicer blade to the machine and shred the yams. Transfer the shredded yams to a large bowl and toss with salt, pepper, garlic and onion, and dried herbs. Heat the fat in a large cast iron skillet over medium heat. When the oil is shimmering, add the seasoned sweet potatoes/yams. Toss everything in the olive oil and cook for a minute. Then, pop on a lid for a few more minutes while the sweet potatoes cook. The hash is ready when there's some crunchy brown bits and texture is soft and tender. Place into serving bowls and top each serving with a sunny side up egg.

51 Tofu Lettuce Wraps

Makes 4 servings.

Organic Ingredients:

- 14 oz package extra-firm tofu, drained and crumbled
- 2 Tbsps. olive oil
- 8 Tbsps. tahini, divided
- 6 thinly sliced green onions), divided
- 1/2 cup plus 2 Tbsps. chopped fresh cilantro, divided
- 3 Tbsps. liquid aminos
- 1 teaspoon grated fresh ginger
- 2 teaspoons honey
- 1/2 teaspoon hot pepper flakes
- 1 cup matchstick-cut cucumbers
- 1 cup matchstick-cut carrots
- 2 cups hot cooked coconut rice (see recipe)
- 8 Bibb lettuce leaves

Simple Preparation:
To prepare filling, spread crumbled tofu in a single layer on several layers of paper towels; cover with additional paper towels. Let stand 20 minutes, pressing down occasionally. Heat a large nonstick skillet over medium-high heat. Add the olive oil to pan; swirl to coat. Add 1/3 cup green onions; sauté 1 minute. Add tofu; sauté for 4 minutes, stirring occasionally. Add 2 tablespoons cilantro, liquid aminos, ginger, honey, and hot pepper flakes; sauté 1 minute. Remove from heat; stir in cucumbers, carrots, and remaining green onions. Spoon 1/4 cup rice and 1 Tbsp. tahini into each lettuce leaf. Top with about 1/2 cup tofu mixture; sprinkle with 1 tablespoon cilantro.

52 Easy Flaked Almond Salad

Makes 6 servings.

Organic Ingredients:

- 1 cup raw almonds, soaked
- 2 celery stalks, finely chopped
- 2 green onions, finely chopped
- 1 garlic clove, minced
- 3 Tbsps. vegan mayo (see recipe)
- 1 teaspoon Dijon mustard
- 1 Tbsp. fresh lemon juice, to taste
- 1/4 teaspoon fine grain sea salt
- black pepper, to taste
- Pinch of kelp granules (optional)
- 1 English cucumber, peeled (if desired) and sliced into 1 cm rounds

Simple Preparation:

Soak almonds in a bowl of water for 3-9 hours until plump. Drain and rinse well. Pour almonds into a food processor and process until finely chopped. It should look a bit like flaked tuna fish. Place into a medium mixing bowl. Add the chopped celery, green onion, garlic, mayo, mustard, and lemon into the bowl. Stir well to combine. Season to taste with salt and pepper. Add a pinch of kelp granules if desired. Slice cucumber into rounds. With a small spoon, gently scoop out the center of each cucumber round to create a small well. Spoon the almond mixture onto each cucumber round. Serve on a platter if you wish. You can also serve it in a pita, with crackers, or on top of a salad. Refrigerate leftover salad for up to 3 days.

53 Butter Beans and Greens

Makes 4 servings.

Organic Ingredients:

- 1 cup brown rice
- 3 Tbsps. olive oil
- 1 cup chard, washed and roughly chopped
- 3 garlic cloves, finely sliced
- 15 oz can butter beans, rinsed and drained
- 1/2 teaspoon cumin seeds

Simple Preparation:
Rinse the rice in cold running water until it runs clear. Bring a large pan of water to the boil, cook the rice for 20-25 mins, then drain. Place a wide, lidded pan over a medium heat with 2 Tbsps. oil. Add the chard, salt and pepper and cook, with the lid on, stirring frequently, until the chard leaves are lightly steamed and wilted, about 4-5 mins. Add the garlic and cook until fragrant, then add the butter beans and cook, stirring, until heated through. Add the remaining oil, then the cumin seeds. Stir until evenly combined and serve over the cooked rice.

54 Broccoli and Green Beans with Toasted Hazelnuts

Makes 3 servings.

Organic Ingredients:

- 1 cup fresh green beans, trimmed
- 1 cup thin-stemmed broccoli
- 1/4 cup blanched hazelnuts, roughly chopped
- 3 Tbsps. olive oil

Simple Preparation:
Bring a large pan of water to the boil. Add the beans and simmer for 1 min, add the broccoli and then cook for 3 mins more until tender. Drain. Meanwhile, heat a large frying pan and gently toast the hazelnuts in olive oil until golden brown. Add the drained vegetables into the frying pan and toss until everything is coated.

55 Lentil and Garbanzo Bean Soup

Makes 8 servings.

Organic Ingredients:

- 2 onions, chopped
- 1 cup chopped celery
- 1 cup of diced carrots
- 2 teaspoons of grated, preferably fresh ginger
- 1 teaspoon minced garlic
- 1 teaspoon garam masala
- 1 teaspoon turmeric
- 1/2 teaspoon ground cumin
- 1/4 teaspoon ground cayenne pepper
- 6 cups vegetable broth
- 1 cup lentils
- 2, 15 oz cans of garbanzo beans
- 2 teaspoons extra virgin olive oil

Simple Preparation:
In a large pot, add the olive oil and the onions over a medium-high heat. You will need to sauté the onions for a few minutes, usually 3 or 4 until they are tender. Add your carrots and celery, cooking for an additional 5 minutes. Stir in your garlic, garam masala, turmeric, cumin, and cayenne pepper and cook for about 40 seconds. Add your vegetable broth and the remaining ingredients and cook until your lentils are tender. This usually takes approximately 90 minutes. To create a thicker soup, take half of it and puree it before stirring it back into the remaining soup.

56 Lentil Soup

Makes 4 servings.

Organic Ingredients:

- 15 oz can lentil beans
- 1 teaspoon olive oil
- 1 onion diced
- 1 carrot chopped
- 4 cups vegetable broth
- 1/4 teaspoon pepper
- 1/4 teaspoon dried thyme
- 2 bay leaves
- 1 Tbsp. lemon juice

Simple Preparation:
Place a strainer in the sink. Open the can of lentil beans and pour them into the strainer. Rinse the beans well until you no longer see bubbles. In a large pot, sauté the onions and carrot in the olive oil for 3 to 5 minutes until onions turn clear. Add the vegetable broth, lentils, pepper, thyme, bay leaves and salt. Reduce heat to a simmer. Cover and cook until the carrots are soft, about 10 minutes. Remove the bay leaves and stir in the lemon juice before serving.

57 Quinoa Cranberry Salad

Makes 4 servings.

Organic Ingredients:

- 1 cup dried quinoa
- 2 cups fresh water
- 1 teaspoon extra virgin olive oil
- 1/2 cups dried cranberries
- 1/2 cup pine nuts
- 2 Tbsps. fresh parsley chopped
- 2 Tbsps. fresh mint chopped
- 1/2 lemon juiced

Simple Preparation:
Bring the water to a boil in a pot on the stove. Add the quinoa. Reduce the heat to a simmer. Place a cover and the pot and cook for 15 minutes. If your quinoa package has cooking instructions on the back, please refer to those instructions. Place your pine nuts is a sauté pan and heat them over medium heat until they are a little toasted. Be careful because they burn easily. In a large bowl combine the cooked quinoa, olive oil, dried cranberries, pine nuts, and parsley, mint and lemon juice.

58 Roasted Vegetable Salad with Garlic Dressing and Toasted Pepitas

Makes 6 servings.

Organic Ingredients:

- 1 medium head garlic
- 4 Tbsps. olive oil
- sea salt and ground black pepper to taste
- 1 bunch carrots, scrubbed
- 1 bunch beets, scrubbed with greens trimmed
- 1 bunch rainbow chard or beet greens
- 1 Tbsp. lemon juice
- 1/3 cup raw, hulled pepitas

Simple Preparation:

Preheat the oven to 350°F and set a large pot of water on the stove and bring to a boil. Cut the root end off of the garlic. Set out a square of foil, drizzle in a teaspoon of olive oil, and a pinch of sea salt. Set head of garlic in the oil and wrap the foil around it. Set foil packet in a small oven-proof dish, and slide into the oven. Bake for 15 minutes and then set aside to cool. Once you remove garlic, turn oven up to 425°F. Meanwhile, peel the carrots. Blanch the carrots in boiling water for 2 minutes, then set aside to cool. Add the beets to the same water used for the carrots. Boil the beets for 8 – 10 minutes, remove with a slotted spoon, and run under cold water. At this point, the skins should readily peel off; use your fingers or a peeler for tougher skins. Halve the carrots and cut beets into quarters or sixths, depending on size. Arrange each on a separate baking sheet {to preserve color}, drizzle each with 1 – 2 teaspoons olive oil and sprinkle with sea salt. Slide into the oven and roast for 15 – 20 minutes, flipping vegetables halfway through. Arrange the chard and beet greens on another rimmed baking sheet. Drizzle with just a touch of oil, rub it all over the leaves and sprinkle with a tiny pinch of sea salt. Slide into the oven and bake for 4 – 6 minutes, or just until leaves have softened. Keep a close eye on these, you just want them to soften and brown slightly. Meanwhile, make the dressing. First, squeeze the roasted garlic out of the papery skin. Set in a small bowl, and mash with a fork. Mix in lemon juice and a pinch of sea salt. Next, whisk in 1 Tbsp. olive oil until mixture is emulsified. Finally, to toast the pepitas, heat a small skillet over medium heat. Add a drizzle of olive oil and the pepitas. Cook, stirring constantly, just until the pepitas start to pop, 1 – 2 minutes. Remove from heat, toss with a little sea salt, and set aside to cool. To serve, toss carrots and beets with the prepared dressing. On a large platter, layer roasted chard on the bottom, topped with carrots and beets, and finish with a drizzle more of dressing, toasted pepitas, a sprinkle of sea salt, and a few twists of black pepper.

59 French Bean Salad

Makes 4 servings.

Organic Ingredients:

- 4 handfuls French beans, stalk ends removed
- 2-3 heaped Tbsps. Dijon mustard, to taste
- 2 Tbsps. balsamic vinegar
- 4 Tbsps. olive oil
- sea salt
- freshly ground black pepper
- 1 medium shallot, peeled and finely chopped
- 1 tablespoon capers, optional
- 1/2 clove garlic, finely grated
- 1 small handful fresh chervil, optional

Simple Preparation:
Bring a pan of water to a fast boil, add your beans, put a lid on the pan, and cook for at least 4 to 5 minutes. Meanwhile, put the mustard and vinegar into a jam jar or bowl and, while stirring, add the olive oil to make a good hot French dressing. Season carefully with sea salt and freshly ground black pepper, then add the finely chopped shallot, the capers if you're using them and the garlic. Remove one of the beans from the pot and drain in a colander. Now, while the beans are steaming hot, this is the perfect moment to dress them – a hot bean will take on more of the wonderful dressing than a cold one. It is best to serve the beans warm, not cold, and certainly not at fridge temperature because the flavors will be muted. Serve the beans in a bowl, sprinkled with chervil if you like.

60 Vegetable Pho

Makes 2 servings.

Organic Ingredients:

- 8 cups vegetable broth
- 6 green onions, thinly sliced
- 1 Tbsp. fresh ginger, peeled and grated
- sea salt to taste
- 2 Tbsps. olive oil
- 6 oz shiitake mushrooms, tough stems removed
- 1 1/2 tablespoon hoisin sauce
- 14 oz brown rice noodles, cooked
- 8 oz bean sprouts
- 2 jalapeño peppers, thinly sliced (optional)
- Fresh cilantro, basil, lime wedges, hoisin sauce for serving.

Simple Preparation:
In a large pot, combine the vegetable broth, green onion, grated ginger, and salt. Bring to a full boil, then reduce the heat and simmer for 15 minutes. While the broth is cooking, heat the olive oil in a pan and add the mushrooms and sauté for about 6 minutes, or until tender, stirring frequently. Stir in the hoisin and sesame oil and cook until the sauce thickens and coats the mushrooms, about 1 minute more. Remove from heat. Divide the rice noodles between four to six large bowls, then fill each bowl with the ginger broth. Add bean sprouts, sliced jalapeños, shiitake mushrooms, fresh basil, and cilantro and serve with lime wedges and hoisin sauce.

61 Garden Soup

Makes 4 servings.

Organic Ingredients:

- 1 medium onion, chopped
- 2 sticks of celery, chopped
- 1 medium leek, chopped
- 2 cloves of garlic, minced
- 2 Tbsps. olive oil
- 2 baby zucchini, peeled and chopped
- sea salt and black pepper to taste
- 4 cups vegetable stock
- 1 cup podded fresh peas
- 1 cups baby spinach, chopped
- a few sprigs of fresh mint

Simple Preparation:

Combine the chopped vegetables in a bowl. Place a large pot on a medium heat and add 2 tablespoons of olive oil. Once hot, add all the chopped vegetables, turn the heat down to low and cook with the lid askew for 10 to 15 minutes, or until tender, stirring occasionally. Once the vegetables are cooked, add the peas or beans and the spinach and cook for a further 4 minutes, or until the peas are tender. Carefully remove the pot to a heatproof surface and leave for a minute or two to stop bubbling. Carefully blitz with an immersion blender until smooth. Pick and roughly chop the mint leaves, discarding the stalks. Carefully ladle the soup into bowls and sprinkle over the mint.

62 Lemon Rice

Makes 6 servings.

Organic Ingredients:

- 2 cups brown basmati rice
- 5 cups filtered water
- 5 Tbsps. olive oil
- 2 Tbsps. mustard seeds
- 2 teaspoons small dried split peas
- 1 handful curry leaves
- rind and juice of 2 lemons
- 1 bunch fresh coriander, chopped
- sea salt
- freshly ground black pepper

Simple Preparation:
In a large pot bring the water to a boil. Add the rice to the boiling water, simmer covered for 40 minutes and drain. Heat the oil in a small frying pan, over a medium heat. Add the mustard seeds and as they begin to pop add the dried split peas, curry leaves and strips of lemon rind (remove these with a microplane). Leave to cook for 1 minute until the dried split peas and lemon peel are lightly colored. Add the drained steaming rice to a bowl and pour over the cooked spices, lemon juice and chopped coriander. Season to taste.

63 Squash and Barley Salad With Balsamic Vinaigrette

Makes 4 servings.

Organic Ingredients:

- 1 butternut squash, peeled, seeded and cut into long pieces
- 1 Tbsp. olive oil
- 1 cup pearl barley
- 1 1/4 cup broccoli, cut into medium-size pieces
- 1 small red onion, diced
- 2 Tbsps. pumpkin seeds
- 1 Tbsp. small capers, rinsed
- 15 black olives, pitted
- 1/8 cup basil, chopped

For the dressing:

- 5 Tbsps. balsamic vinegar
- 6 Tbsps. olive oil
- 1 Tbsp. Dijon mustard
- 1 garlic clove, finely chopped

Simple Preparation:
Heat oven to 400°F. Place the squash on a baking tray and toss with olive oil. Roast for 20 mins. Meanwhile, boil the barley for about 25 mins in salted water until al dente. While this is happening, whisk the dressing ingredients in a small bowl, then season with salt and pepper. Drain the barley, then tip it into a bowl and pour over the dressing. Mix well and let it cool. Boil the broccoli in salted water until just tender, then drain and rinse in cold water. Drain and pat dry. Add the broccoli and remaining ingredients to the barley and mix well. This will keep for 3 days in the fridge and is delicious warm or cold.

64 Lentil and Wild Rice Salad

Makes 4 servings.

Organic Ingredients:

- 1 cup dry wild rice
- 1 cup edamame
- 1 cup lentils
- 1 cup loosely packed chopped cilantro
- 1/2 cup broken almonds
- 1 Tbsp. apple cider vinegar
- 2 Tbsps. fresh lemon juice
- 1 teaspoon grated fresh ginger
- 1 Tbsp. liquid aminos
- 3 Tbsps. extra virgin olive oil

Simple Preparation:
Cook the wild rice in 1 1/4 cup of water for time on package (about 50 minutes). Drain and cool. Boil the lentils for about 20 minutes (you don't want them too soft and mushy). Drain and cool. Cook or thaw the edamame according to the instructions on the package. Whisk together in a bowl the apple cider vinegar, lemon juice, ginger, Bragg's Liquid Aminos and olive oil. Place the wild rice, lentils, edamame, nuts and cilantro into the bowl and toss with your dressing. Enjoy!

65 Thai Coconut And Mushroom Soup

Makes 4 servings.

Organic Ingredients:

- 2 Tbsps. Thai red curry paste
- 3 cloves garlic, minced
- 2, 14 oz cans coconut milk
- 1 1/2 cups not-chicken stock
- 1 carrot, shredded into matchsticks
- 8 oz baby bella mushrooms, lightly rinsed and sliced
- 4 cups baby spinach
- juice of 1-2 limes (to taste)
- 1/2 teaspoon liquid aminos
- coarse salt and freshly ground pepper
- 1/2 cup cilantro leaves, plus more for garnish

Simple Preparation:
Bring a large pot over medium-high heat. Add the curry paste and press it into the pot, releasing the oils. Do this for about a minute. Add the garlic and 1/3 cup coconut milk and stir to combine and bloom and become fragrant. Then add the rest of the coconut milk and not-chicken stock. Then add the carrot and mushrooms. Let simmer about 5 minutes, until everything is heated through. Add the spinach to wilt. Take it off the heat and squeeze in lime juice, along with the liquid aminos. Add the cilantro and salt if needed. Serve garnished with cilantro.

66 Pumpkin Soup

Makes 8 servings.

Organic Ingredients:

- 1 cup chopped onion
- 1-inch piece of ginger, peeled and minced
- 1 clove garlic, minced
- 6 cups vegetable stock, divided
- 4 cups pumpkin puree
- 1 teaspoon sea salt
- 1/2 teaspoon chopped fresh thyme
- 1/2 cup almond milk
- 1 teaspoon chopped, fresh parsley

Simple Preparation:
In a large pot over medium high heat, cook onions, garlic and ginger in 1/2 cup of the vegetable stock. Continue cooking until completely tender. Approximately 5 minutes. Add the pumpkin, remaining stock, sea salt and thyme. Cook for an additional 30 minutes. Using a handheld blender, puree the soup until it look completely smooth. Remove your soup from the heat and add the milk. Top with parsley and serve. If you want a thicker soup, mix in a little chia seed powder.

67 Broccoli Dal

Makes 6 servings.

Organic Ingredients:

- 1 Tbsp. oil
- 1 onion, diced
- 3 cloves garlic, minced
- 1 cup broccoli
- 1 cup red lentils
- 3 cups vegetable stock
- 1/2 teaspoon curry powder
- 1/4 teaspoon garam masala
- black pepper
- sea salt

Simple Preparation:
Heat the oil in a saucepan, and add the onion and garlic. Cook over a medium heat for a few minutes, stirring occasionally, until the vegetables are fairly soft. Meanwhile, add the broccoli to a food processor, and blend until no large chunks remain. When the onion is soft, add the processed broccoli and lentils to the pan, along with the stock and spices. Mix well, and bring to a simmer. Cook gently, stirring regularly, until the lentils are cooked and the mixture reaches the desired consistency - around 20-25 minutes. Serve warm with brown rice

68 Black Bean Cauliflower Salad

Makes 4 servings.

Organic Ingredients:

- 1 1/2 cups wild rice
- 2 Tbsps. olive oil
- 1 teaspoon cumin
- 1 small red onion, thinly sliced
- 1 Tbsp. turmeric
- 1 clove garlic, finely chopped
- 2 Tbsps. fresh ginger, grated
- 1 head cauliflower, cut into bite-sized pieces
- 15 oz can cooked black beans, drained and rinsed
- 1 Tbsp. agave nectar
- 3 Tbsps. chopped fresh cilantro

Simple Preparation:

In a pan over medium heat, heat the olive oil and cumin together for 1 minute. Add the onion, turmeric and sauté for 6 minutes, or until the onions are caramelized. Add the garlic and half of the ginger and cook these ingredients for 1 minute. Add the cauliflower and cover the pan. Reduce the heat to medium-low and cook for 6 minutes. Add black beans and heat for 1 minute. Remove the pan from the heat and add the remaining ginger and the agave nectar. Garnish your dish with cilantro.

69 Quinoa-Stuffed Acorn Squash Rings

Makes 4 servings.

Organic Ingredients:

- 2 Tbsps. olive oil
- 1/2 cup quinoa, rinsed thoroughly
- 1 cup vegetable broth
- 1 medium onion, diced
- 1 apple, cored and diced
- 1/4 cup dried cranberries
- 2 Tbsps. chopped sage
- 2 Tbsps. chopped walnuts
- salt and pepper to taste
- 1 egg, whisked
- 3 small acorn or sweet dumpling squash, cut into 1/2-inch slices (remove seeds)
- 1 Tbsp. honey

Simple Preparation:
Preheat oven to 375°F. Coat two cookie sheets with oil and place squash rings on sheets. Cook quinoa in the vegetable broth according to package directions. Cool slightly. Heat the olive oil in a medium skillet over medium heat. Add onion. Cook about 10 minutes, or until onion is just beginning to brown. Add apple and cook about 5 minutes more, until apple is softened. Allow to cool slightly. Combine quinoa, apple and onion mixture, cranberries, sage, and walnuts in a large bowl. Add salt and pepper to taste. Stir in egg. Brush tops and insides of squash rings with honey; season with salt and pepper. Stuff quinoa filling into the center of each squash ring, pressing down to fit as much stuffing as possible without overflowing. Bake 30-40 minutes, or until tops are golden brown and squash is tender.

70 Barley Chickpea Salad

Makes 6 servings.

Organic Ingredients:
For the salad:

- 1 cup barley
- 1/4 cup pine nuts
- 1 leek, finely diced
- 3 Tbsps. olive oil
- juice of 2 lemon
- 1/8 cup raisins
- 15 oz can chickpeas, drained
- 4 Tbsps. chopped fresh herbs such as parsley, mint and coriander

To serve:

- Mixed greens
- Radish
- Celery sticks

Simple Preparation:
Cook the barley according to packet instructions. Allow to cool. Lightly toast the pine nuts in a non-stick pan over a low heat, until golden. Put all the salad ingredients into a bowl and toss together well. Taste and adjust the seasoning if necessary. Serve piled on to plates or into bowls with mixed greens, radishes and celery.

71 Vegetable Curry

Makes 4 servings.

Organic Ingredients:

- 1 medium red onion, peeled and chopped
- 2 Tbsps. olive oil
- 1 zucchini, diced
- 1/2 butternut squash, peeled and diced
- 1/2 cup mushrooms, quartered
- 1 red pepper, diced
- 1 cup cauliflower, broken into florets
- 2 1/2 cups curry base sauce (see below)
- 1 2/3 cups filtered water

Simple Preparation:
In the olive oil, cook the onion gently for 10 minutes in a large pan then add the remaining vegetables and stir together. Add the curry base sauce and simmer gently for around 25 to 30 minutes, taking care not to overcook the vegetables. If the sauce becomes too thick, add a little water to achieve the desired consistency.

72 Sugar Snap Pea and Carrot Soba Noodles

Makes 4 servings.

Organic Ingredients:
Soba:

- 6 oz brown rice soba noodles
- 2 cups frozen edamame
- 10 oz (about 3 cups) sugar snap peas or snow peas
- 6 medium-sized carrots, peeled
- 1/2 cup chopped fresh cilantro (about 2 handfuls)
- 1/4 cup sesame seeds

Ginger-sesame sauce:

- 1/4 cup reduced-sodium tamari or soy sauce
- 2 Tbsps. olive oil
- 1 small lime, juiced
- 1 Tbsp. honey or agave nectar
- 1 Tbsp. white miso
- 2 teaspoons freshly grated ginger
- 1 teaspoon chili garlic sauce

Simple Preparation:
To prepare the vegetables, slice the peas in half lengthwise (or just roughly chop them). Slice the carrots into long, thin strips with a julienne peeler, or slice them into ribbons with a vegetable peeler. To make the sauce: whisk together the ingredients in a small bowl until emulsified. Set aside. Bring two big pots of water to a boil. In the meantime, toast the sesame seeds: Pour the sesame seeds into a small pan. Toast for about 4 to 5 minutes over medium-low heat, shaking the pan frequently to prevent burning, until the seeds are turning golden and starting to make popping noises. Once the pots of water are boiling: In one pot, cook the soba noodles just until al dente, according to package directions (about 5 minutes), then drain and briefly rinse under cool water. Cook the frozen edamame in the other pot until warmed through (about 4 to 6 minutes) but before draining, toss the halved peas into the

boiling edamame water and cook for an additional 20 seconds. Drain. Combine the soba noodles, edamame, snap peas and carrots in a large serving bowl. Pour in the dressing and toss with salad servers. Toss in the chopped cilantro and toasted sesame seeds.

73 Coconut Curry

Makes 4 serving.

Organic Ingredients:
For the Curry:

- 1 Tbsp. olive oil
- 1 small onion, diced
- 4 cloves garlic, minced
- 1 Tbsp. fresh grated ginger (or 1 tsp ground)
- 1/2 cup broccoli florets (or green bell pepper), diced
- 1/2 cup diced carrots
- 1/3 cup snow peas (loosely cut)
- 1 Tbsp. curry powder
- pinch cayenne (optional for heat)
- 2, 15 oz cans light coconut milk
- 1 cup veggie stock
- Sea salt and black pepper

For the Coconut Quinoa:

- 14 oz can light coconut milk
- 1 cup quinoa, rinsed in a fine mesh strainer*
- 1 Tbsp. agave nectar (optional)

For Serving:

- Fresh lemon juice, cilantro, mint and/or basil, red pepper flake

Simple Preparation:
If serving with coconut quinoa, begin by washing thoroughly in a fine mesh strainer. Add to a medium saucepan over medium heat and toast for 3 minutes. Add 1 can light coconut milk and 1/2 cup water. Bring to a boil, then reduce heat to simmer, cover and cook for 15 minutes or until the quinoa is light, fluffy and the liquid is absorbed. Set aside until serving. In the meantime, heat a large saucepan or pot

to medium heat and add 1 Tbsp. coconut oil. Add the onion, garlic, ginger, carrot, broccoli and a pinch each salt and pepper and stir. Cook, stirring frequently, until softened – about 5 minutes. Add curry powder, vegetable stock, coconut milk and stir. Bring to a simmer then reduce heat slightly and continue cooking for 10-15 minutes. Add the snow peas in the last 5 minutes so they don't overcook. Taste and adjust seasonings as needed. Serve over coconut quinoa and garnish with fresh lemon juice and herbs.

74 Curry Base Sauce

Makes 2 servings.

Organic Ingredients:

- 1/2 cup red lentils
- 2 medium onions, peeled and roughly chopped
- 3 medium carrots, roughly chopped
- 2 Tbsps. olive oil
- 6 cloves garlic, peeled and roughly chopped
- 1/3 cup fresh ginger, peeled and roughly chopped
- 6 stalks coriander, chopped
- 1 Tbsp. ground coriander
- 1 Tbsp. ground cumin
- 1/2 teaspoon ground black pepper
- 1 Tbsp. ground cinnamon
- 1 Tbsp. turmeric
- 1 Tbsp. garam masala
- 1 1/3 cups filtered water
- 1 cup coconut milk
- salt and freshly ground black pepper

Simple Preparation:
Wash the lentils, then place them in a pan and cover with cold water. Bring to the boil and simmer gently for 15 to 20 minutes, or until tender. Meanwhile, blend all the vegetables, garlic and ginger in a food processor until finely chopped. Heat enough oil to cover the bottom of a large saucepan, put it on a low heat, add the spices and cook gently for a couple of minutes. Then add the onions, carrots, pepper, garlic, ginger, coriander stalks, the chili and all the spices and cook gently for 5-10 minutes until the onions start to soften. Add the water and lentils and simmer for another 30 minutes before adding the coconut milk. Bring to the boil then remove from the heat and blend until smooth using an immersion blender. Season to taste. Set aside to cool then use as required.

75 Asian Mushrooms with Wild Rice

Makes 4 servings.

Organic Ingredients:

- 1 1/2 cups wild rice
- 3 Tbsps. olive oil
- 1 large onion, diced
- 12 oz assorted fresh Asian mushrooms, trimmed and sliced
- 1/4 teaspoon dried thyme
- 1/4 cup apple cider vinegar
- 1/4 cup fresh water
- 1/2 cup chopped fresh flat-leaf parsley

Simple Preparation:
Cook the wild rice in 4 1/2 cups of water for time on package (about 50 minutes). Drain and cool. Meanwhile, pour the olive oil in a pan on medium heat; add the diced onion, and sauté 7 minutes or until golden. Add your Asian mushrooms and sauté 4 to 5 minutes or until mushrooms are tender. Add the dried thyme, the apple cider vinegar and water, and sauté 3 minutes or until the liquid is absorbed. Stir the mushroom mixture and parsley into your prepared rice. Enjoy!

76 Roasted Root Veggies with Quinoa

Makes 4 servings.

Organic Ingredients:

- 1 bag baby carrots
- 1 bunch parsnips, cleaned and cut into baby carrot sized pieces
- 1 white onion, chopped into cut into baby carrot sized pieces
- 1 box vegetable broth (approximately 4 cups)
- 2 Tbsps. extra virgin olive oil
- 1 cup quinoa

Simple Preparation:
Heat the oven to 400°F degrees. Spread the carrots, parsnips and onion out in a flat layer on a baking sheet. Pour the olive oil over the top of the vegetables and mix it around to coat the vegetables. Place the baking sheet in the oven and set the timer for 40 minutes. We want the vegetables to be cooked and just starting to turn golden – not burnt, so baking times may vary depending on your oven's intensity. Bring the vegetable broth to a boil in a pot on the stove. Add the quinoa. Reduce the heat to a simmer. Place a cover and the pot and cook for 15 minutes. If your quinoa package has cooking instructions on the back, please refer to those instructions. Place the cooked quinoa into an individual serving bowl and cover it with your cooked root vegetables.

77 Hearty Dream Bean Stew

Makes 8 servings. Vegan and Kosher for Passover.

Organic Ingredients:

- 2 cups dried butter beans
- 4 cups or 1 box vegetable broth (see below)
- 4 cups filtered water
- 4 cups diced carrots
- 4 cups diced cauliflower
- 2 cups dried quinoa
- 15 sprigs fresh thyme
- 2 large bay leaves
- sea salt and black pepper to taste

Simple Preparation:
Fill a large soup pot with the water and the vegetable broth. Bring to a boil. Add the dried beans, cover the pot and cook for 90 minutes. Make sure that there is always plenty of water in the pot. Add carrots, cauliflower, thyme and bay leaves and cook for 20 minutes. Then add the quinoa and cook for an additional ten minutes. Add salt and pepper to taste.

78 Vegetable Broth

Makes 8 cups.

Organic Ingredients:

- 1 Tbsp. olive oil
- 3 large onions, quartered
- 2 large carrots, quartered, tops reserved
- 8 large garlic cloves, crushed
- 2 large leeks, washed, trimmed, tough outer leaves removed
- 1 large sprig thyme
- 1 large sprig rosemary
- 1 bay leaf
- 6 whole black peppercorns
- 1 whole clove
- 3 quarts water

Simple Preparation:
Preheat oven to 400°F. In a large bowl toss the oil with onions, carrots, garlic, leeks and arrange them in a roasting pan. Place pan in oven and roast, stirring once, for 45 minutes or until golden brown and tender. In a large pot combine the roasted vegetables with carrot tops, thyme, rosemary, bay leaf, peppercorns, clove and water. Bring to a boil, reduce heat and simmer, stirring occasionally for 1 hour or until the broth is reduced to about 8 cups. Strain. Optional Ingredients: celery root, parsley root, dried sage, summer squash, green beans, marjoram, oregano, or mushrooms (dried or 1 pound fresh).

79 Quinoa Stuffed Portabella

Makes 8 servings.

Organic Ingredients:

- 1 medium yellow onion, finely chopped
- 2 Tbsps. olive oil
- 1/2 cup finely chopped celery
- 1 cup vegetable broth
- 2 cloves of minced garlic
- 1 Tbsp. ground cumin
- 10 oz chopped spinach
- 2 cups water
- 15 oz can black beans, rinsed and drained
- 3/4 cup quinoa
- 3 large carrots, grated
- 4 large portabella mushrooms, washed and stems removed

Simple Preparation:
Heat the olive oil in a saucepan over medium heat. Add the onion and celery and cook for 5 minutes or until completely tender. Add the cumin and garlic and sauté for about 1 minute. Stir in the spinach. Cook for 5 more minutes or until the liquid has evaporated. Stir in the black beans, quinoa, carrots, and 2 cups of water. Cover and bring to a boil before reducing heat to medium-low. Simmer for an additional 20 minutes, or until the quinoa has become tender. Season with salt and pepper if desired. Preheat the oven to 350F and add the vegetable broth to the bottom of a baking dish. Fill each of your portabella caps with a heaping amount of the quinoa mixture and place them onto the baking dish. Cover with foil and bake for approximately a half hour. Remove the foil and bake for approximately 10 minutes more. Let stand for 5 to 10 minutes and transfer to serving dishes. Top with chives or parsley if desired.

80 Roasted Summer Vegetables and Chickpeas

Makes 8 servings.

Organic Ingredients:

- 5 baby zucchini, peeled and thickly sliced
- 3 garlic cloves, chopped
- 5 carrots, peeled and chopped into sticks
- 1 onion, chopped
- 1 Tbsp. coriander seeds
- 4 Tbsps. olive oil
- 14 oz can chickpeas, rinsed and drained
- 2 cups vegetable broth
- small bunch cilantro, roughly chopped

Simple Preparation:
Heat oven to 430°F. Pour all the vegetables into a large roasting pan and toss with the coriander seeds, most of the olive oil and salt and pepper. Spread everything out to a single layer, then roast for 45 minutes, tossing once or twice until the vegetables are roasted and brown round the edges. Place the pan on the stovetop on a low heat, then add the chickpeas and vegetable broth. Bring to a simmer and gently stir. Season to taste, drizzle with olive oil, then scatter over the cilantro. Serve with mashed black beans (see below).

81 Mashed Black Beans

Makes 4 servings.

Organic Ingredients:

- 1 Tbsp. olive oil
- 3 crushed garlic cloves
- 2, 15 oz cans black beans, rinsed and drained

Simple Preparation:
Heat olive oil in a large frying pan. Add garlic and cook for 1 min, stirring all the time. Add black beans. Season and cook for 2 minutes.

82 Hot and Sour Soup

Makes 6 servings.

Organic Ingredients:

- 2 cloves of garlic
- sea salt and white pepper
- 1 inch piece of ginger, minced
- 1 cup shiitake mushrooms, cleaned
- 1 cup bamboo shoots, drained
- 2 Tbsps. olive oil
- 2 Tbsps. liquid aminos
- 2 Tbsps. apple cider vinegar
- 1 teaspoon honey
- 6 cups hot vegetable stock
- 14 oz firm tofu
- 2 spring onions, chopped
- 1/2 bunch of chives
- 1 large egg (optional)

Simple Preparation:

Heat the olive oil in a large wok or heavy-based saucepan over a medium-high heat, add the mushrooms and cook for 4 minutes, or until lightly golden. Stir in the garlic, ginger, salt and bamboo shoots and cook for a further minute. Meanwhile, mix together 3 Tbsps. of liquid aminos, 4 Tbsps. of apple cider vinegar, the honey and a good pinch of white pepper. Stir the mixture into the pan and cook for a minute, then pour in the hot stock and bring gently to the boil. Reduce the heat to low and simmer for 10 minutes, or until slightly reduced. Meanwhile, chop the tofu into 1/2 inch cubes and whisk the egg well. Once reduced, remove the soup from the heat. Using a chopstick, stir the soup in a clockwise direction until you get a little whirlpool, then slowly add the beaten egg, stirring continuously to form thin ribbons. Stir in the tofu and return to the heat for 1 minute to warm through. Season to taste, then serve immediately with the spring onions and chives scattered on top.

83 Bean and Pesto Mash

Makes 6 servings.

Organic Ingredients:

- 1 Tbsp. olive oil, plus a drizzle to serve (optional)
- 2, 15 oz cans cannellini beans, rinsed and drained
- 2 Tbsps. pesto (see below)

Simple Preparation:
Heat the oil in a large saucepan. Add the beans and cook for 3-4 mins until hot through. Lightly mash with a potato masher for a chunky texture. Stir through the pesto and season. To serve, drizzle with a little olive oil, if you like.

84 Pesto Sauce

Makes 1 cup.

Organic Ingredients:

- 2 cups packed fresh basil leaves
- 2 cloves garlic
- 1/4 cup pine nuts
- 2/3 cup extra-virgin olive oil, divided
- Kosher salt and freshly ground black pepper, to taste

Combine the basil, garlic, and pine nuts in a food processor and pulse until coarsely chopped. Add 1/2 cup of the oil and process until fully incorporated and smooth. Season with salt and pepper. If using immediately, add all the remaining oil and pulse until smooth. If freezing, transfer to an air-tight container and drizzle remaining oil over the top. Freeze for up to 3 months.

85 Turmeric Tofu and Wild Rice

Makes 4 servings.

Organic Ingredients:

- 1/2 cup wild rice
- 1 1/2 cups filtered water
- 2 Tbsps. olive oil
- 14 oz medium to firm tofu
- 1/4 teaspoon turmeric
- 1 teaspoon soy sauce

Vegetable stir-fry:

- 1 teaspoon coconut oil
- 1 small onion, long thin slices
- 1/2 clove garlic
- 1/4 teaspoon Himalayan salt
- 3/4 cups carrots, chopped
- 3/4 cups broccoli, chopped
- 2 Tbsps. liquid aminos
- Garnish: coriander, lime, salt, black pepper

Simple Preparation:
Place the tofu on a kitchen towel to soak up excess water for 5-10 minutes. To cook the wild rice, boil the rice and water in a pan on low heat for around 40 minutes until the rice grains are soft and cooked. While the rice is cooking, chop the tofu in small cubes and place in a separate pan with the olive oil on low heat so that they become slightly brown. Add the turmeric and soy sauce to the tofu after 5-10 minutes, sprinkling over all the tofu pieces, and turn the tofu so that all the sides become brown, careful not to break them. You can start the vegetable stir-fry while the tofu is still cooking. Place the coconut oil and onion slices in a large pan and let this cook on low heat for a few minutes before adding the chopped or grated garlic. Once cooked, add the carrots and broccoli and stir. Let this cook for 7-10 minutes before adding the cooked rice. You can now stir in the liquid aminos and add the tofu. Serve with a slice of lime and a sprinkle of salt, coriander and black pepper.

86 Layered Squash and Barley Spinach Pie

Makes 6 servings.

Organic Ingredients:
For the filling:

- 1 small butternut squash, peeled, seeded and cubed
- 3 Tbsps. olive oil, plus a little extra for brushing
- 3 onions, finely chopped
- 3 garlic cloves, crushed
- 1/2 cup mushrooms, sliced
- 1/2 cup whole cooked chestnuts, quartered
- 1/2 cup pearl barley
- 5 1/2 cups vegetable stock
- 1 Tbsp. liquid aminos
- zest of 1 lemon
- 1 oz pack of fresh sage, leaves picked and chopped
- 1 2/3 cups baby spinach
- 1 oz pack parsley, leaves chopped

Raw cauliflower crust (see below)

Simple Preparation:
Heat oven to 400°F and roast the butternut squash with 1 Tbsp. oil for 25-30 mins until tender, then set aside. Meanwhile, heat remaining oil in a large pan and cook the onions and garlic for 10 minutes until soft. Remove two-thirds, then add the mushrooms, chestnuts and pearl barley to the pan. Sizzle for a few mins, pour in the stock, and then bring to the boil. Boil for 30 mins until the barley is tender and sticky and there is no liquid left. Stir in the liquid aminos, season and set aside. While the barley layer is cooking, make the other layers. Stir the zest and a good amount of seasoning into the reserved onions until smooth. Take a third of the mixture and gently fold with the sage and roasted squash. For the final layer, boil the kettle, then pour half the spinach into a large colander. Pour over the boiling water to wilt, then repeat with the rest of the spinach. Pour the spinach onto a clean tea towel and squeeze out all the moisture you can. Roughly chop, then mix into the mixture with the parsley. To make the pie,

brush a 4 cup false bottom bread loaf pan with a little olive oil. Make 3 long triple layer strips of foil and lay these across the width of the tin to help you lift out the pie to serve. Press a cauliflower crust into the bottom of the bread loaf pan, pressing evenly into the corners and sides. Spoon in the spinach layer, smooth the surface, then repeat with the barley and finally the squash layer. Dome the squash mix slightly to give a rounded top. Roll out the remaining cauliflower crust to fit then press the lid over the top. Can be covered and chilled overnight. Heat oven to 400°F and put a large baking sheet inside. Brush the surface of the pie with egg, place onto the heated baking tray and bake for 30 mins, then reduce the heat to 350°F and bake for a further 1 hour until the top is golden brown and feels hard. Stand for 15-20 minutes and serve.

87 Cauliflower Crust

Makes 1 crust.

Organic Ingredients:

- 1 head cauliflower
- 2 whole eggs
- 4 Tbsps. of coconut flour
- 1 Tbsp. garlic powder
- 1 Tbsp. sea salt
- 1 Tbsp. dried basil
- 1 Tbsp. dried oregano
- 1 Tbsp. fresh ground black pepper

Simple Preparation:

Preheat oven to 350°F. To create the pureed cauliflower, simply chop all the cauliflower florets into small pieces, place it into a blender and blend until pureed. Place the cauliflower puree into a cheesecloth sheet over a large bowl (to catch the liquid) and squeeze the excess water from the cauliflower. Let the cauliflower sit within the cheesecloth for about 5 minutes, returning to squeeze any further water. Discard the cauliflower liquid. The end result will resemble a firm puree. Combine the remaining ingredients into a large bowl and hand mix until thoroughly combined. Spread the "dough" into either 1 large pizza shape or 2 small pizza rounds on a parchment paper covered cookie sheet about ¼ inch thick. Bake at 350°F for about 20 minutes, then place another sheet of parchment paper on top of the crust to help you flip the crust without breaking it. Cook the crust until the top is golden brown and firm to touch. If you're making a pizza, take the crusts out of the oven and top with your favorite toppings. Bake for another 10-15 minutes at 400F or until everything on the top has warmed and melted.

88 Sundried Tomato Basil Pasta

Makes 4 servings.

Organic Ingredients:

- 2 cups brown rice pasta, macaroni shaped
- 6 cups filtered water
- 1 cup fresh basil leaves
- 2 cups sundried tomatoes, dry
- 2 stalks green garlic, white part only - not the tough leaves, chopped
- 4 cloves garlic, pressed through a garlic press
- 1/2 yellow onion, diced
- 1 Tbsp. dried oregano
- 4 Tbsps. olive oil
- 1 Tbsp. honey
- 1 Tbsp. sea salt

Simple Preparation:
Bring the water to a boil. Place the sundried tomatoes in a small dish. Pour just enough boiling water into the dish to cover the tomatoes, and let sit for 10 minutes. Pour the brown rice pasta into the boiling water and cook according to the directions. Brown rice pasta turns mushy faster than regular pasta, so you should check it about 2 minutes before you think it will be done. Strain the cooked pasta and rinse under cold water. Set aside. Pour your rehydrated sundried tomatoes into a food processor with the basil, dried oregano and 2 Tbsps. olive oil. Process until smooth. In a hot frying pan add 2 Tbsps. olive oil, the onion, green garlic, and regular garlic. Cook carefully, stirring constantly to avoid burning the garlic. When the edges start to turn brown, and the honey and continue cooking until everything in the pan is golden brown. Combine the pasta with the sundried tomato sauce and browned garlic. Season to taste with sea salt.

89 Sunflower Seed Risotto

Makes 4 servings.

Organic Ingredients:

- 2 Tbsps. olive oil
- 2 onions, diced
- 2 celery sticks, diced
- 2 leeks, diced
- 1 cup crimini mushrooms, diced
- 1 bunch thyme, tied together
- 1 1/2 cups sunflower seeds
- 2 cups vegetable stock
- 1 cup peas, frozen
- sea salt and pepper
- 4 Tbsps. toasted almond slivers

Simple Preparation:
In a large pot add the olive oil and cook the onions, leeks, celery and mushrooms until turning brown at the edges. Then add a small amount of vegetable stock, just to wet the bottom of the pot to keep the vegetables from sticking. Tie the thyme with a rubber band and place in the pot with the vegetables. Add sunflower seeds to the pot once the vegetables are golden then cover with vegetable stock. Be careful not to add too much stock, it needs to come just to the top of the seed mix. Bring everything to a boil, place a lid on top and turn heat down to a simmer. Let cook for at least an hour or until the seeds are tender. Puree a third of the cooked ingredients add to the rest of the mix. Add the frozen peas and cook until they are hot. Season with salt and pepper and top with toasted almond slivers.

CHAPTER 4
Sweet Treats

Everyone knows that, when you diet, you're going to miss a few things. You're going to want dessert and treats and we all know that fruit, while delicious, sometimes just doesn't cut it when it comes to getting that special treat. So what are your options? I've listed a few.

1 Chocolate Chia Pudding

Makes 4 servings.

Organic Ingredients:

- 1 1/2 cups unsweetened almond milk
- 1/3 cup chia seeds
- 1/4 cup cacao
- 3 Tbsps. agave syrup
- 1/2 teaspoon ground cinnamon
- 1/4 teaspoon sea salt
- 1/2 teaspoon pure vanilla extract

Simple Preparation:
Add all ingredients except sweetener to a mixing bowl and whisk vigorously to combine. Sweeten to taste with the agave syrup. Let rest covered in the fridge overnight or at least 1 hour until it's achieved a pudding-like consistency. If blending, add to a blender and blend until completely smooth and creamy, scraping down sides as needed. Leftovers keep covered in the fridge for 2-3 days, though best when fresh. Serve chilled with desired toppings, such as fruit coconut whipped cream.

2 Strawberry Lime Mango Crisp

Makes 6 servings.

Organic Ingredients:
Crisp Topping:

- 1/4 cup melted virgin coconut oil
- 1/4 cup applesauce
- 1/8 teaspoon pure stevia extract powder
- 1 cup shredded unsweetened coconut
- 1/2 cup quinoa flakes
- 1/2 cup chopped almonds
- 1 teaspoon ground dried ginger
- 1/2 teaspoon ground cardamom
- 1/4 teaspoon ground or freshly grated nutmeg
- pinch unrefined salt

Filling:

- 4 cups chopped fresh mangos
- 2 cup fresh strawberries
- 1 1/2 Tbsps. lime zest
- 1 Tbsp. fresh lime juice
- 2 Tbsps. arrowroot starch
- 1 Tbsp. grated fresh ginger root
- 1/16 teaspoon/pure stevia extract powder

Simple Preparation:
Pre-heat oven to 375°F, and lightly oil a 10-inch round baking dish. In a small bowl, toss together ingredients for topping until mixture is evenly moistened and mixed. Set aside. In a large bowl combine mango, strawberries, lime juice, lime zest, and ginger. Sprinkle in stevia and starch, and lightly toss. Transfer fruit mixture into prepared baking dish. Sprinkle topping evenly over the top of the fruit. Bake for 40 minutes, until fruit is bubbling and topping is browned. Allow to cool for at least 30 minutes before serving. Store leftovers covered in the refrigerator.

3 Vegan Pumpkin Cheesecake

Makes 8 servings.

Organic Ingredients:
Crust:7

- 1 3/4 cups toasted almonds, ground
- 5 Tbsps. coconut oil, melted

Cheesecake:

- 12 oz package of firm silken tofu, gently pressed dry
- 1 1/2 Tbsps. olive oil
- 1 3/4 cup pumpkin puree
- 2 teaspoon pumpkin pie spice
- 2/3 cup unsweetened almond milk
- 1/4 cup honey
- 2 Tbsps. arrowroot powder
- 2 Tbsps. fresh lemon juice

Simple Preparation:
Preheat oven to 350°F and add toasted almonds to food processor and mix until a fine meal is achieved (alternatively, smash with a rolling pin in a large freezer bag). Add melted coconut oil and pulse to combine. Transfer to a standard 9 inch pie pan and press down with your fingers to form the crust evenly on the bottom and up the sides of the pan. Bake for 11 minutes or until slightly browned, then set aside to cool. Keep oven at 350°F. In the meantime, prepare cheesecake filling by adding all ingredients to a blender and blending until creamy and smooth, scraping down sides as needed. Taste and adjust seasonings/sweetness as needed. Pour cheesecake filling into pre-baked crust and bake at 350°F for 1 hour. The edges should be golden brown and the center should be slightly jiggly. Let cool completely, then loosely cover with a paper towel (to catch moisture) and then very loosely with foil and chill for at least 6 hours or overnight before serving. Store in the fridge for up to a 3 days.

4 Double Chocolate Cookies

Makes 16 servings.

Organic Ingredients:

- 2 large eggs
- 1 cup raw unsalted creamy almond butter
- 1 teaspoon vanilla extract
- 1/2 teaspoon apple cider vinegar
- 12 drops liquid stevia
- 1/2 cup honey
- 1/4 cup unsweetened cocoa powder
- 2 tablespoons buckwheat flour
- 1/2 teaspoon baking soda
- 1/4 teaspoon sea salt
- 1/4 cup unsweetened shredded dried coconut

Simple Preparation:
Preheat oven to 350°F. Line 2 cookie sheets with parchment paper. Beat eggs with an electric-mixer in a medium bowl and then add almond butter, vanilla, apple cider vinegar, honey and liquid stevia. Do not mix the rest of the wet ingredients together. Mix the dry ingredients in a separate large bowl - unsweetened cocoa powder, buckwheat flour, baking soda, sea salt and dried coconut. Combine the wet and dry ingredients and mix well with an electric-mixer until thoroughly mixed. At first it will seem too dry, but keep mixing and it will form into a thick, fudge-like dough. Finish mixing with a spatula to make sure it is well mixed. Then evenly drop the dough onto a cookie sheet. Flatten the cookies gently using the back of a spoon or your fingertips. Bake for about 12 minutes, they will still be gooey and moist on the inside. Cook less when in doubt, they firm up as they cool.

5 Pumpkin Oatmeal Squares

Makes 6 servings.

Organic Ingredients:

- 1 flax egg (1 tablespoon ground flax mixed with 3 tablespoons water)
- 1/2 cup unsweetened canned pumpkin purée
- 3/4 cup coconut flavor
- 1 teaspoon pure vanilla extract
- 1/2 teaspoon baking soda
- 1/2 teaspoon fine grain sea salt or pink Himalayan sea salt
- 1 1/2 teaspoons cinnamon
- 1/2 teaspoon ground ginger
- 1/8 teaspoon ground nutmeg
- 3/4 cup gluten-free rolled oats, ground into a flour (Or use 3/4 cup + 1 tablespoon oat flour)
- 3/4 cup gluten-free rolled oats
- 3/4 cup almond flour (not almond meal)
- 1 Tbsp. arrowroot powder (for enhanced binding)
- 1/2 cup pecan halves, chopped
- 2 Tbsps. mini non-dairy chocolate chips, for garnish

Simple Preparation:
Preheat oven to 350°F and line an 8-inch square pan with parchment paper. Mix flax egg in a small bowl or mug and set aside to thicken for about 5 minutes. In a large mixing bowl, beat the pumpkin and coconut flavor with electric beaters until combined. Pour in the flax egg and vanilla extract and beat until combined. Add the baking soda, salt, cinnamon, ginger, and nutmeg and beat again. Finally add in the oat flour, rolled oats, almond flour, arrowroot flour, and pecans. Beat until combined. Spoon dough into prepared pan and spread out until smooth and even. The dough will be very sticky, but this is normal. I like to cover the dough with a piece of parchment paper and roll it with a pastry roller. Sprinkle the chocolate chips on top and press down. Bake for 18 minutes, until lightly golden and firm to the touch. Be sure not to over bake. Place pan on a cooling rack for 10 minutes. Then, lift out and place square directly on cooling rack for another 10-20 minutes, until cool. Slice and enjoy! The bars will crumble slightly if sliced warm, but they firm up nicely when cooled.

6 Coconut Whipped Cream

Makes 2 cups.

Organic Ingredients:

- 14 oz can coconut cream
- 1 Tbsp. honey
- 1 teaspoon vanilla extract
- 5 drops vanilla stevia
- pinch of sea salt

Simple Preparation:
Chill your coconut cream or milk in the fridge overnight. Also chill a large mixing bowl 10 minutes before whipping. The next day, remove the can from the fridge without tipping or shaking and remove the lid. Scrape out the top, thickened cream and leave the liquid behind (reserve for use in smoothies). Place the cream in your chilled mixing bowl. Beat for 30 seconds with a mixer until creamy. Then whip in the honey, vanilla extract, stevia, and salt. Use immediately or refrigerate - it will harden and set in the fridge the longer it's chilled. Will keep for up to 1 - 2 weeks.

7 Granola Cluster Cookie Bites

Makes about 2 dozen 2-inch cookies.

Organic Ingredients:

- 9 Medjool dates, pitted
- 3/4 cup agave syrup
- 1 teaspoon vanilla extract
- 1/4 cup coconut oil, liquefied
- 1 1/2 cups oats or quinoa flakes
- 1 1/2 cups blanched slivered almonds
- 2/3 cup almond flour
- 1 1/2 Tbsp. coconut flour
- 1/4 cup roasted cocoa nibs or chocolate chips (optional)

Simple Preparation:
Preheat oven to 350°F. Line large baking sheet with parchment paper. Chop dates fairly well. Add chopped dates to large mixing bowl and add agave syrup and vanilla extract. Stir so that the date pieces are covered. Set aside. Toast the oats (or quinoa flakes) and nuts. Add coconut oil, oats (or quinoa flakes), nuts, and all other ingredients to the mixing bowl that you set aside earlier. Mix until all ingredients are incorporated. Let batter sit for at least 5 minutes or so until it thickens and "sets up" naturally. Drop dough by rounded tablespoonful onto prepared baking sheet. Use your fingers to press batter into mounds if necessary. The cookies can be placed close together as they will not spread when baked. Bake for about 12 minutes until cookies are set and fairly golden brown. Cool on baking sheet another minute or two. Remove with spatula to cool.

8 Almond Pecan Scones

Makes 8 scones.

Organic Ingredients:

- 1/2 cup raw pecans
- 1/2 cup raw almonds
- 1/2 cup rolled oats
- 2 cups barley flour
- 3 teaspoons baking powder
- 1 teaspoon cinnamon
- 1/4 teaspoon sea salt
- 1/3 cup unsweetened applesauce
- 1/3 cup agave syrup plus 2 tablespoons for topping
- 2 Tbsps. coconut oil, melted
- 1 Tbsp. vanilla flavoring
- 1/4 cup chopped pecans or almonds

Simple Preparation:
Preheat oven to 375°F. Line a cookie sheet with parchment paper. Place first 3 ingredients in a food processor and process until mixture becomes a meal and no chunks remain. Transfer to a large mixing bowl and combine with the rest of the dry ingredients. In a small bowl mix together the wet ingredients then add to the dry ingredients and fold in nuts. Mix together until it forms a firm dough ball. I usually use my hands toward the end. Sprinkle a little flour onto the parchment paper and transfer the dough to the sheet. Gently press the dough into an 8-inch circle then cut into 8 pieces with a sharp knife. You do not need to separate the wedges. Glaze the tops with 2 Tbsps. agave syrup. Bake for 15-20 minutes. Slightly cool then transfer to a cooling rack. Great alone or served with a sugar free all fruit apricot blueberry compote.

9 Almond Granola Bars

Makes 4 servings.

Organic Ingredients:

- 1 1/2 cups rolled oats
- 1 cup brown rice crisp cereal
- 1/2 cup sliced almonds
- 1/4 cup unsweetened shredded coconut
- 2 Tbsps. chia seeds
- 1/4 cup coconut oil, melted
- 1/2 cup roasted almond butter
- 1/4 cup agave nectar syrup
- 1 teaspoon real vanilla extract
- pinch of fine grain sea salt or pink Himalayan salt, to taste
- 1 1/2 Tbsp. mini very dark sugar free chocolate chips

Simple Preparation:
Line an 8-inch or 9-inch square pan with two pieces of parchment paper, one going each way so it's easy to lift out. In a large bowl, stir together the oats, brown rice crisp cereal, sliced almonds, coconut, and chia seeds. In a medium pot over low heat, melt the coconut oil. Remove from heat and stir in the almond butter, agave nectar, and vanilla, until smooth. Pour wet mixture over dry and stir well until thoroughly combined. Add a pinch of salt to taste and stir again. Spoon mixture into the pan and roughly spread out (but don't pack down yet). Sprinkle on the very dark chocolate chips in an even layer. Wet hands lightly and then press down the mixture until even. Use a pastry roller to roll it out and pack it in even more. Transfer pan to the freezer for about 10 minutes until firm. Slice into bars, wrap, and store in the fridge or freezer. These bars fall apart easily so I don't recommend leaving them at room temperature for longer than a few minutes.

10 Pumpkin Pie

Makes 6 serving.

Organic Ingredients:
For the Crust:

- 1 cup of almonds, finely ground in blender until flour-like
- 3 Tbsps. of coconut oil plus some to grease pie pan
- 1 egg
- 1/2 teaspoon cinnamon

For the Filling:

- 15 oz can of pumpkin
- 3 eggs
- 1/4 cup of honey
- 1 Tbsp. of pumpkin pie spice
- 1 teaspoon natural vanilla
- coconut milk to thin (no more than about 1/3 cup)

Simple Preparation:
Grease a pie pan with coconut oil and mix crust ingredients by hand in a medium sized bowl. Press crust into bottom and sides of pie pan and put in the oven while making the filling. In the same bowl combine the filling ingredients (except coconut milk) and mix using an immersion blender. If you don't have one of these, use a regular blender or food processor. A hand-mixer will not get it as smooth! It should be smooth and spreadable, but not really pourable. Add coconut milk if needed to thin slightly. After 10-15 minutes, remove the crust as it barely starts to brown. Pour/smooth the filling over the crust and return to oven for about an hour or until center is no longer jiggly. Will set more as it cooks. Top with coconut whipped cream.

11 Brownies

Makes 9 servings.

Organic Ingredients:

- 1 cup of almond butter
- 1 1/2 cup zucchini, shredded in a food processor
- 1/3 cup of honey
- 1 egg
- 1 teaspoon of vanilla
- 2 teaspoons of arrowroot starch
- 1 teaspoon of cinnamon
- 1/2 teaspoon of nutmeg
- 1 cup of very dark sugar free chocolate chips, melted

Simple Preparation:
Preheat oven to 350°F degrees. Combine all the ingredients into a large bowl and mix everything together. Pour into a greased 9×9 baking pan. Bake for 35-45 minutes or until a toothpick comes out clean.

12 Baked Bananas

Makes 1 serving.

Organic Ingredients:

- 1 banana
- 1 Tbsp. almond butter
- 1/2 teaspoon cinnamon

Simple Preparation:

Preheat your oven to 375°F degrees. Using a butter knife, cut about 1/2 inch deep down the length of the banana. With the back of a spoon, widen the cut to make room for the almond butter. Spoon the almond butter throughout the opening in the banana. Sprinkle with cinnamon. Wrap completely in aluminum foil. Bake for 15 minutes. Remove from oven and let cool for 1-2 minutes. Unwrap and either eat directly from the foil or move to a plate.

13 Plantain Crepes

Makes 4 servings.

Organic Ingredients:

- 2 medium plantains, light green or yellow with spots is fine (pureed 1 1/2 cups)
- 4 eggs
- 1/2 cup water
- 1/4 cup coconut oil, melted + more for cooking crepes

Filling: sliced banana, honey, sea salt

Simple Preparation:
Peel and roughly chop plantains and puree in food processor until really smooth and all chunks removed. Add remaining ingredients and blend well. Heat a 9-10 inch skillet over medium-low heat. Brush with coconut oil. Add about 1/4 cup crepe batter to pan and swirl in an even layer around the pan. These crepes need to be cooked for a longer temperature on lower heat. Don't try to turn until they are nice and brown. Use a very thin spatula to gently get underneath the crepe to flip without tearing it. They will only need to cook on the other side about 1/4 the time of the first. Fill with sliced bananas, honey and a pinch of sea salt.

14 Crunchy Coconut Apples

Makes 2 servings.

Organic Ingredients:

- 1 1/2 cups coconut flakes
- 2 Tbsps. cacao powder
- 1 Tbsp. cacao nibs
- 1 1/2 teaspoons cinnamon
- 1/8 teaspoon nutmeg
- 1/4 cup agave syrup
- 1 organic green apple sliced

Simple Preparation:

In a medium sized mixing bowl add coconut flakes, cacao powder, cacao nibs, and cinnamon, nutmeg and agave syrup. Stir well, for 2-3 minutes, until the maple syrup is fully combined and the dry mixture starts to turn wet from the syrup. Clean and dry the apple. Thinly slice the apple starting from the outside and working your way toward the center. Repeat on the other side. Then lay the apple flat on one of the cut sides and chop thin slices of the remaining sides of the apple core. Transfer the sliced apple to a serving tray. Pour the cocoa-nut mixture on top of each apple. Now you can serve them right away or let them sit for an hour or longer to let the coconut flake mixture soften.

15 Honey Nut Bars

Makes 6 servings.

Organic Ingredients:
Crust:

- 1 1/2 cups almond flour
- 7 Tbsps. coconut oil, melted
- 1 Tbsp. raw honey
- pinch of salt

Topping:

- 1 cup raw almonds
- 1/2 cup raw cashews
- 1/2 cup raw macadamia nuts
- 1/3 cup raw cacao nibs
- 3 Tbsps. raw honey
- 3 Tbsps. olive oil
- 2 Tbsps. coconut milk, full fat
- 2 teaspoons vanilla extract
- 1/4 teaspoon ground cinnamon

Simple Preparation:
Mix the ingredients for the crust and press the dough into the bottom of an 8x8-inch pan lined with parchment paper. Gently heat the honey, olive oil and coconut milk in a saucepan, stirring frequently. Remove from heat and mix in the pure vanilla extract and ground cinnamon. Add the nuts and cacao nibs to the honey mixture and stir together until fully coated. Refrigerate mixture for 20 minutes, stirring once after 10 minutes. Spread the nut mixture evenly on top of the crust and bake at 350°F for 20 minutes or until nuts start to turn brown on the edges. Allow the pan to cool on a wire rack and refrigerate until set. Store in an airtight container in the fridge.

16 Lemon Bars

Makes 12 servings.

Organic Ingredients:
Crust:

- 4 cups almond flour
- 1/2 cup arrowroot starch
- 1/2 teaspoon salt
- 1/2 cup honey
- 2 teaspoons pure vanilla extract
- 1 cup coconut oil, melted

Lemon Topping:

- 4 eggs
- 3/4 cup honey
- 1/2 cup lemon juice
- 1 Tbsp. lemon zest
- 5 Tbsps. arrowroot starch

Simple Preparation:
Preheat oven to 325°F and grease a 9×13 pan with coconut oil. Combine all ingredients in a large bowl, then press into the greased 9×13 pan. Bake in oven for about 30 minutes, until golden brown. To make the lemon topping, beat together all ingredients. Let crust cool for about 15 minutes, and when crust is ready, pour lemon topping over crust (note: it will be liquid), then bake another 20 minutes or so, until set. For best results, chill before eating.

17 Strawberry Cheesecake Bars

Makes 4 servings.

Organic Ingredients:

- 1 cup finely ground toasted almonds, plus more for garnish
- 1 heaping cup soaked raw cashews (soaked overnight or at least 4 hours)
- 1/2 cup peeled and diced zucchini
- 1/4 cup coconut oil, melted
- 2 Tbsps. canned coconut milk, full fat, room temperature
- 2 Tbsps. pure agave syrup
- 4 Tbsps. honey
- 1/2 Tbsp. pure vanilla extract
- 1/8 teaspoon sea salt
- juice of one and a half lemons, separated
- 1 cup fresh organic strawberries, hulled and diced

Directions:

Divide the cup of finely ground almonds into the bottom of 4 (8-ounce) glasses and set them aside. In a high-powered blender, process the raw cashews until they are blended. Add the zucchini, coconut oil, coconut milk, agave syrup, 2 Tbsps. honey, vanilla extract, salt, and the juice of one lemon. Add lemon juice as needed to your preference. Then blend again until a super smooth and creamy batter is formed. Pour the cheesecake batter evenly into the 4 (8-ounce) glasses leaving some room for the strawberry sauce. Place them in the freezer and allow them to set for at least an hour or longer. While the cheesecake is setting go ahead and make your strawberry sauce. In a heavy bottomed sauce pot over medium-high heat, add the juice of half a lemon, the strawberries, and honey. Mash the strawberries together until they are combined with the rest of the ingredients. Let the mixture boil and reduce, stirring intermittently, for about 10-12 minutes or so. Once the mixture has reduced and thickened remove from heat and set aside. When your cheesecake is ready, remove mason jars from the freezer, let thaw for about 15 minutes before serving. Top with strawberry sauce. Garnish with fresh strawberry slices and a sprinkle of almonds.

18 Chocolate Mousse

Makes 6 servings.

Organic Ingredients:

- 1 ripe avocado
- 1/4 cup date paste or 4 medjool dates, pitted
- 1 Tbsp. honey
- 1 cup full fat coconut milk
- 1/2 cup organic cacao powder
- 1/4 teaspoon Ancho Chili powder (optional)
- 1/4 teaspoon Himalayan salt
- 1 Tbsp. pure vanilla extract

Simple Preparation:

Process avocado, date paste (or pitted medjool dates), honey and coconut milk in a small food processor until smooth and creamy. Add cacao powder, ancho chili powder, salt and vanilla and resume processing until well incorporated. You might have to scrape the sides once or twice to get all the powder to mix in nicely. Transfer this mixture to the bowl of your stand mixer and whisk on high for 4-5 minutes until light and fluffy. You could also do this with a hand mixer if you don't have a stand mixer. Divide the chocolate mousse between 6 individual dessert bowls, dust lightly with cacao powder or ancho chili powder and refrigerate for 4-6 hours, or up to 2 days. Note that this mousse can also be served immediately, but its texture greatly benefits from it sitting in the fridge for at least a few hours.

CHAPTER 5
Whole Week Grocery Shopping

When it comes to grocery shopping, you must remember that everyone is different. There is a chance that you just don't like kale or can't stand blueberries. That's fine. This is just a guide and a way to direct you in the right direction. If nothing else, you should understand that your body is always right. Listening to it can help you through the adjustment process and help you make the right decisions at mealtime.

My primary advice in this category is not to shop while you're hungry. Temptation can get the better of you. You have to fight to maintain your health and remember all the work you've put into achieving your goal.

Keep in mind, again, that this is just a guide and my sample shopping list is just an example. How many snacks you want is a personal preference, and how many times you want to eat salad or substitute a wrap is a personal preference. Adding to it, or making a few alterations here and there is fine. Just remember to watch out for those sneaky sources of sugar.

THE VITALITY DIET: THE VEGETARIAN/VEGAN ANTI-INFLAMMATORY

Organic items I always keep stocked in our kitchen:

- Extra-virgin, cold-pressed California olive oil
- Coconut oil for baking and higher heat cooking
- Raw honey from a local beekeeper
- Agave nectar
- Oat, Almond, Garbanzo bean, Brown Rice flours
- Aged Balsamic Vinegar
- Apple Cider Vinegar
- Sea Salt
- Black Peppercorns in a grinder
- Dried herbs and spices like: cumin, thyme, curry, cinnamon, turmeric, nutmeg, carob powder, oregano, etc.
- Brown Rice
- Quinoa
- Oats
- Black Beans
- Garbanzo Beans
- Unsweetened Almond or Soy Milk
- Fresh Fruits and Vegetables
- Eggs

Shopping List for an Entire Week

- Brown Rice
- Eggs
- Unsweetened Almond and Soy Milk
- Black Beans
- Garbanzo Beans
- Onions
- Garlic
- Mixed Greens
- Sweet Potatoes
- Asparagus
- Broccoli
- Spinach
- Apples
- Blueberries
- Raspberries
- Quinoa
- Carrots
- Almonds

Again, don't get stingy with the vinegar and olive oil quality.

Have fun with your diet. Don't forget that. And above all, don't forget that with every day that passes not only are you going to feel better, but you're going to look better. And most of all, you're going to be a lot healthier for it.

REMEMBER: NOTHING TASTES AS GOOD AS BEING HEALTHY AND ATTRACTIVE FEELS!

Please contact me with any questions. My email address is:
Sarah@Manski.org

Disclaimer:
The material in this book is simply an introduction to the anti-inflammatory diet. This book is not intended to serve as a prescription for you or to replace the advice of your medical doctor. Please discuss all aspects of the anti-inflammatory diet with your physician before beginning the program. If you have any medical conditions, or are taking any prescription or nonprescription medications, see your physician before altering or discontinuing your use of medications.

The fact that a website or another source is listed in this book as a potential source of information does not necessarily mean that I or the publisher endorse information it may provide or recommendations it may make.

Nothing in the title or content of this book is intended to suggest that the use of the anti-inflammatory diet is a guarantee you will be cured of illness. The evidence, carefully presented in this book, substantiates that the nutritional regimen recommended is very frequently effective in losing weight and maintaining health. Even so, I offer no guarantee that every individual will benefit from the anti-inflammatory diet.

Made in the USA
Las Vegas, NV
26 October 2021